Disclaimer: The presented information in this book is solely meant for educational purposes. The content presented is to the best knowledge of the author. This book does not intent to replace the evaluation or treatment by a medical professional. Before following any advice, the reader is encouraged to conduct their own research in partnership with a health care professional.

This book is dedicated to my beloved husband who encouraged me to write it in the first place. He supported and motivated me throughout the process.

Also, Roman Fessler, thank you for your availability to answer any of my questions throughout my writing process. Your fasting institute and the lessons you teach make a true difference to people's lives.

Table of Contents

1. Introduction

1.1 My discovery of fasting

The first article I came across on fasting was many years ago and focused on intermittent fasting. Back then my main goal was to lose weight and according to the information I found online, all you had to do is fast for 16 to 20 hours and you would shed pounds! The times I did stick to eating during my designated eating windows, not snacking in between meals and keeping 16 to 18 hours meal-free I did lose weight successfully. But as you might have figured, it worked only when I stuck to all those things. My progress halted as soon as I allowed myself a little snack or coffee with milk.

I went as extreme as eating only once a day which I realized soon did me no good and was not sustainable. Since my stomach had shrunken so much, it became a struggle to get all my nutrients in from one meal. I would end up forcing myself to eat beyond my stomach size or under-eat and being hungry soon after. Over the years I saw how gradually but consistently my weight crept up. It was only about one pound a year but I felt like the progression was unstoppable.

I was frustrated and felt like I didn't know how to kick-start healthy eating habits. That was until a fateful conversation in the summer of 2019. My dad owns a bar and throughout my adolescent years, I have helped out there. It is a small business with many locals and regular customers, so personal conversations were often part of the work. Many of the regulars were middle-aged men, single (often divorced) and from all classes of society. One of these men was Robert. He is in his mid-40s and divorced with four children. He is one of the kindest people I have ever met and I always enjoyed hearing about his personal life. We got along from the very beginning and he would refer to me as one of his daughters because, in fact, his second oldest daughter and I are the same age. A series of unfortunate events led to him being physically limited. It all started when he slipped at a spa and injured his knee. During surgery he contracted multi-resistant bacteria. Due to the many follow-up surgeries, he started to compensate for the limitation in his knee which led to other problems. He had to get surgery on one side of his hip, then the second knee and finally also on the other side of his hip. This left him unable to walk on his own and he needs crutches now, as well as a mix of drugs to deal with the aftermath of all the surgeries. In order to allow his body to detox from the medication cocktail, he goes once a year on a 10-day fast at "Heilfasteninstitut Fessler" (*heilen* means *to heal* in German, *fasten* is *to fast* and *Institut* is the same word in English *institute*) in the countryside of Austria. These fasts are referred to as therapeutic fasts or fasting cures. When he first told me about paying money to be starved – technically, he is given teas, soups, smoothies and some supplements – I laughed it off as a ridiculous waste of money. At the same time, when he mentioned the significant weight loss, I was intrigued. I researched it and found a variety of places offering extended fasts. Some allowed for a fast from home, others offered shorter fasts at fancy resorts. I went back to Robert with my newly acquired knowledge and quizzed him about what was so special about this Roman Fessler, the founder of "Heilfasteninstitut

Fessler" and why it has to be ten days (not five, not seven not 14 but ten days). He outlined some aspects and I decided to give it a try. Ever since, I am convinced of the health benefits of extended fasts, or *cures* as some call them, and the self-healing powers of your body. As a side-effect, you lose weight and it becomes easy to manage the new weight.

This book will cover the background and history of fasting, with a focus on extended fasts, undisclosed research from the former Soviet Union, recent scientific revelations and finally the Roman Fessler method for successful and long-term weight loss and health.

1.2 Background and history

Most people associate the abstinence of food with weakness. Allow me to start off this chapter by giving you some examples of what in fact is possible in a fasted state.

Paul Bragg, an American alternative health food advocate and fitness enthusiast, described in his book "The Miracle of Fasting" (1967) his trek through Death Valley in California while completely fasting – and that in the heat of the summer. He walked 30 miles in two days of the desert's scorching heat. At the same time, a group of young athletes, not restricting themselves in food, could not walk 15 miles on the same path.

In 1965 a group of healthy men aged 17 to 53 years walked 50 km (31 miles) per day over ten days to get from Stockholm to Gothenburg in a fasted state. They drank 2.7 liters of water every day. Five of them observed their weight during the trip and saw a weight loss of 9 kg each (approx. 19.84 lbs.), of which 5 kg (11 lbs.) constituted fat, 3 kg (6.6 lbs.) water and 1 kg (2.2 lbs.) protein. Their physical condition was considered overall good.

A similarly successful event was reported in Moscow in 1981 when three men and three women, all in good health, aged 19 to 57 years conducted a 19-day long trekking trip in the Moscow region. Under medical supervision, they covered 538 km (334.3 miles) out of which 406 km (252.3 miles) were completed during a complete water fast.

As a more extreme example the surgeon Moiseev does an annual 30-day fast. While fasting, he continues his professional work and participates in surgical operations.[1]

Today's living conditions promote many illnesses: diabetes, hypertension (high blood pressure), obesity, cancer. As a result, prescription drug consumption is shooting through the roof. However, side effects of many pharmaceuticals come with their own risks. Common drug treatments today have their own limitations. All over the globe fasting is being researched as a form of therapy and cure.[2]

Throughout history, fasting has been part of human life. The willful abstinence from food, drink, or both for health, religious, ceremonial or ethical purposes has been practiced from antiquity to present by medical practitioners, members of religions, culturally nominated individuals (e.g. hunters or candidates for initiation rites), and individuals using it as a form of protest against violations of social, ethical or political principles.

Unwillingly, humans had to go through long periods of no access to food or water due to famine, food insecurity or shortages of drinking water which forced an evolutionary adaptation. Only in recent years has the human body experienced constant food supply and the problems that come with it.

1.2.1 Historical medical application

Have you ever experienced the loss of appetite when you were sick? Most people are raised to eat when they are sick, even when their intuition tells them not to. The so-called fasting instinct has not always been recognized by physicians. This instinct naturally signals the patient in certain disease states to abstain from food by experiencing a loss of appetite.

It is believed that fasting has been used therapeutically since at least the 5th century BCE. The Greek physician Hippocrates recommended abstinence from food or drink for patients who exhibited certain symptoms of illness. Administering food during these stages was believed to be unnecessary, sometimes even detrimental, since fasting was thought to be an important natural part of the recovery process.

The first organized studies of fasting were carried out in animals and humans in the late 19th century and substantially contributed to the first understanding of the physiological effects fasting can have on the organism. Methods of fasting evolved in the 20th century, with the understanding of nutrition and nutritional requirements of the human body becoming known. A wide range of methods developed. Physicians realized that fasting can be used in disease prevention or as a form of treatment.

Various settings were used to promote fasts for example in a hospital, clinic or at home. The treatment of chronic diseases foresaw at times month-long fasts and consumption was reduced to water and calorie-free tea. It included light exercise and enemas; the latter being considered an important part of cleaning the bowl and re-establishing a healthy gut flora. Another method was developed: the modified fast. It allowed for consumption of up to 500 kilocalories per day, depending on sex, age and activity level. The calories were consumed from bread, vegetable broth, fruit juice, honey or milk. Sometimes it included psychological or spiritual therapy since some people experience spiritual enlightenment, clear thinking and psychological breakthroughs on extended fasts. Soon modified fasts aimed at inducing substantial weight loss. This further evolved into intermittent fasting which cycles between periods of eating and fasting for a certain number of hours or days.[3]

The 21st century brought more clarity: many studies in animals and humans were conducted and research papers released. One research paper, published in 2021, shows that fasting diets could harm the health of future generations. The study shows that reduced food intake in roundworms has detrimental effects on three generations of offspring, especially when those descendants have access to unlimited food. Can findings from ringworms be transferred to humans? It will take many more years to tell.[4]

The medical community is split: while it was clearly established that in certain instances, such as acute diseases (in particular when accompanied by the loss of appetite), fasting was beneficial to human health, in other instances it remained questionable. A closer look will have to be taken.

1.2.2 Religious fasting

Some form of fasting is deeply rooted in many religions. During special sacred times, worshipers abstain from eating and drinking, as a sort of cleanse.

In ancient religions fasting was a practice to prepare worshipers or priests and priestesses to approach deities. The pre-Columbian peoples of Peru, dating back to 10,000 BCE, required fasting as one form of demonstrating penance for sins confessed to a priest or priestess. In other cultures, the practice was considered a way to appease upset deities or aid in resurrecting them when it was believed they had died. Some Native American tribes fasted in pursuit of a vision. The Evenks, an indigenous tribe of Siberia, believed that its shamans received visions after unexplained illness, rather than seeking a vision. Once the initial vision was received, however, they trained themselves to see more visions and control spirits in a fasted state. The spirit-filled religion of the indigenous peoples of the American Southwest, known as the Pueblos, fasted during retreats before major ceremonies connected with seasonal changes.[5]

In the ancient Indian religion of Jain, fasting is undertaken throughout the year and accompanied by designated periods of prayers and meditation, in which the latter can lead in certain cases to trances that enable individuals to disassociate themselves from the world and reach a transcendent state. The members of the tiny faith of Jainism made headlines in 2015, when India's Supreme court considered to ban the practice of santhara or sallekhana which literally means *thinning out*; a tradition where a person who is very old or ill decides to stop eating in order to die. By allowing it, does this constitute assisted suicide?[6]

Buddhist monks of Theravada, the only remaining school from the Early Buddhist period, include fasts as a part of their meditation practice and self-development.

In Zoroastrianism, an ancient pre-Islamic religion of Iran, fasting is prohibited. They believe that such form of abstinence and self-denial for the purpose of spiritual discipline does not strengthen believers in their fight against evil. All other major Western religions, Christianity, Islam and Judaism, practice fasts during certain periods of time. Christians fast, for example during Lent, a 40-day period of prayer and fasting beginning on Ash Wednesday and ending at sundown on the Saturday before Easter. In Islam a full month of fasting is observed every year. During Ramadan, a period of penitence, Muslims fast from dusk until dawn. Judaism has six fasting days each year, with Yom Kippur, the Day of Atonement, being the most significant. On Yom Kippur people of Jewish faith practice forgiveness of the sins of others and genuine remorse for one's own sins against God. Other than that, Jews observe four fasts for mourning purposes.[7]

As you can see, fasting has a long-standing tradition for many people around the globe. What might have been disguised as a religious reason, could actually be rooted in being beneficial.

2. The science behind fasting

Let me start off by explaining what makes a fast a fast. In order to be in a fasted state, it requires a person to not chew on food so that the digestive system can be shut off, as well as, to not trigger the release of insulin, meaning your blood sugar cannot rise above a certain level (depending on exercise level, potential insulin sensitivity and some other factors, this value varies from person to person). Insulin's job is to deliver glucose inside the cell. It takes the ingested glucose, goes from cell to cell, knocks at its door and asks if it needs energy. If a cell needs energy, insulin is the key to open the cell for glucose to enter. If there is glucose left at the end of the run, it will be stored in the liver. This is the reason why modified fasts can be effective as long as the juices and soups consumed do not exceed a certain number of calories.

REMEMBER: modified fasts are fasts that allow for the consumption of more than water, up to 500 calories per day in liquid form.

Later in the book, I will explain the energy usage in the body and how it changes when fasting. In this next chapter I will dwell on some of the research that is currently available on fasting.

2.1 The Nobel-Prize-winning discovery of autophagy

In 2016 the Nobel Assembly at Karolinska Institute awarded the Nobel Prize in Physiology or Medicine to Dr. Yoshinori Ohsumi, a Japanese cell biologist, for his discovery of the mechanisms for autophagy. Autophagy stems from the Greek words *auto* meaning *self* and *phagien* meaning eat; the process of "self-eating". What seems at first glance like a self-destructive process, actually is the body's ability to degrade and recycle cellular components for energy. In the process of "self-eating" cellular waste, the cell is provided with nutrients and building blocks for renewal.

Most tissues in the organism regularly replace their cells with new ones. This begs the question, though, of what happens to the dead cells?

Autophagy was first taken up in the 60s when the Belgian biochemist Dr. Christian de Duve examined some liver tissue and observed the existence of recycling compartments, the so-called lysosomes. Lysosomes have special digestive enzymes which help to consume worn-out or damaged tissues, food particles, invading bacteria and viruses. It can go as far as the self-destruction of a cell, if cell damage is beyond repair.

It was not clear, though, how the cell got rid of larger protein complexes and worn-out organelles. Organelles are a subcellular unit that performs specific functions within a cell. Among the more important cell organelles we have the nucleus, which stores the cell's DNA, the mitochondria, which produce chemical energy and ribosomes, which assemble proteins.

The cell garbage is recycled into new cells and energy by the lysosomes and it helps to decompose different protein structures into amino acids. This is later used to create new cells.

Dr. Ohsumi built on Dr. de Duve's findings and showed in his research how autophagy, by degrading and recycling cellular components, provides fuel for energy and building blocks for renewal of cellular components. It is an essential surviving tool for the cell's response to starvation and other forms of stress. When infected with a bacteria or virus, for example, autophagy can eliminate the intruder. However, autophagic activity seems to decrease with age. The cell's functioning deteriorates due to the accumulation of damaged protein and organelles over time and the body becomes more susceptible to illnesses.

In organisms with impaired autophagy, a person can develop type 2 diabetes, Parkinson's disease, even cancer and other age-related disorders. If your natural recycling mechanism does not function properly, damaged cells and other byproducts of tissue renewal start to accumulate in the body and as a result your body becomes incapable of neutralizing cancer cells and cells infected by dangerous viruses and bacteria.

Dr. Ohsumi found that autophagy can be induced by a variety of stressors. A major incentive is calorie restriction or fasting.[8]

This gives you the basis to understand that fasting is not just a religious practice, trend, or the newest alternative lifestyle but actually can provide for a better and healthier life.

2.2 The Russians

Up until the collapse of the Soviet Union, fasting cures were an integral part of the Russian healthcare system. The basis for this unique approach are some findings completely unknown to the west. Thousands of patients took part in a huge study that stretched over four decades. The results are groundbreaking.

THE PRESENT

Our first stop takes us to Sanitarium Goryachinsk. The village is located approximately 110 miles north-east of Ulan-Ude, and about six hours south to the Mongolian boarder. It is known for its hot springs and sand beaches; and since 1751 for being the first health resort on Lake Baikal at the creek "Goraychiy" (meaning *hot* in Russian).[9] Since 1995 a designated building is reserved for therapeutic fasting. Costs for the therapy were reimbursed in the former Soviet Union.

Often patients find the Sanatorium after they received modern treatment at a hospital. However, these treatments are not successful. Therapeutic fasts are a universal method, and welcomed alternative, that can be used with many diseases. Depending on your issue, the length of the fast is adapted. It is followed by a gradual refeeding phase in which calories are carefully increased and solid foods are re-introduced into the diet. The importance of safely restoring the digestive and motor function of the gastrointestinal tract cannot be stressed enough.

Disregard for a gradual return to solid foods can lead to adverse outcomes and in some cases even lead to death.[10]

One such tragic incident was recorded in February 1977 in Moscow when the 39-year-old artist P. followed the recommendation of some healer and decided to conduct a 40-day fast without medical supervision. The fast did not killed him – he managed the 40 days well – it happened that he died two days later. The cause of death was reported as acute heart failure as a result of severe stomach bloating due to ingestion of a large amount of food after prolonged fasting.[11]

Similar stories were told about concentration camp survivors: in some incidents the freed prisoners who had been starved for extended periods of time, passed away from over-eating and their stomachs not being able to digest food anymore.

The therapy in Goryachinsk itself is fairly easy: water, water and more water. The average treatment is twelve days. The duration varies based on the severity of the illness and can last up to three weeks. With chronic ailments, prescription drugs can be discontinued after two to three days. The crucial factor is that the patients fast under medical supervision. No one should attempt to fast on their own – care and support are essential.

In fact, no particular nutritional deficiency occurs while fasting. During the fast, the number of certain vitamins like vitamin C, D and E and some other metabolic products can go slightly down. However, this is not a matter of critical values. The sanitarium treated over 1,000 patients suffering from diabetes, asthma and hypertension to rheumatism and allergies. After undertaking one or multiple fasting cures, 2/3 of patients reported that all symptoms were gone.[12]

FASTING CRISIS

What people struggle with most during the fast is seemingly not the deprivation of food. The sensation of hunger is not noticeable in most cases after two to three days. What makes the fast challenging is the so-called fasting crisis. It is offset by the body switching from using glycogen as a source of energy to fat; your body's reserves. While going through the detox process, fasting people can experience a range of symptoms: irritability, weakness, body aches, headaches, fatigue, difficulty concentrating, outbreak of sweat, skin problems, disturbed sleep, nausea, depressive mood and slightly raised temperature.[13]

The duration and peak of the crisis can be determined through a urinalysis. Due to the food depravation, the pH-value of the blood increases. Sometimes the crisis is accompanied by the patience's disease. For example, if you have a patient that often suffers from headaches, he or she might experience headaches during the fasting crisis. If you have a patient who suffers from gout or arthritis, he or she can experience joint pain. However, this pain does not last longer than 24 to 36 hours. This seems to be the price to pay for the radical change.[14]

The fasting crisis occurs most times after two to five days. Going through a fasting crisis is, in fact, a good sign of your organs working hard to get rid of toxins. It is also considered one of the most important phases during the healing process. Once the worst is overcome – mainly after the fourth or fifth day – most people experience better mood, clearer thinking, sometimes even personal breakthroughs or spiritual enlightenment.[15,16]

WAYS TO PREVENT SEVERE DETOXIFICATION SYMPTOMS

There are methods to prevent severe symptoms of a fasting crisis. For instance, change to a vegan and alkaline diet approximately a week before, or even sooner if possible. In addition, combine this with exercise and drinking a lot of water. Often extended fasts are used to refrain from other everyday vices like sugar, caffein and nicotine. A couple days before the fast, start reducing the intake of these substances. The idea is to reduce the over-acidity in your organism.[17]

I mentioned briefly earlier that the body normally uses glycogen as fuel and during a fast has to use its reserves. Let's look into the sources that are in fact available to our organism.

THE BODY'S 3 ENERGY SUPPLIERS

Before we immerse in the topic, let's briefly look at the difference between glucose and glycogen. Glucose is the sugar that is already roaming through your blood and that is used as the imminent energy source. Glycogen is the stored form of energy. When you eat more sugar than your body needs, the excess will be stored as glycogen in your liver. Your brain primarily operates on glucose.

REMEMBER: Previously the role of insulin was explained in connection with blood sugar and the liver. In order to get into a fasted state, it is crucial to not trigger the release of insulin otherwise your body will not switch from using glycogen to fat as fuel.

Normally your body can live off the glucose in your bloodstream and as the next source will tap into your glycogen reserves which will be reversed into glucose. When you fast, however, these reserves are used up within 24 hours. The next step will be to produce glucose from protein, meaning mainly from the muscles. At the same time the lipid reserves, your fat stores, are used now. The new energy supplier is called ketone or ketone bodies. To recap: when there is not enough glucose for energy in your system, the body produces ketones in the liver, the central organ for metabolic functions. By switching from glucose to fat, it shifts the metabolism into the next gear. Your system is sped up. The opposite happens when calories are too drastically reduced: your metabolism will slow down and start preserving energy.

Cleansing procedures play an important role in fasting. Evidence shows that during longer periods of forced food deprivation, both people and animal often die from the body's self-poisoning by the products of decaying tissues.[18] Voluntary short-term fasts, on the other hand, are not affected by these products if conscious cleansing procedures are in place.

A number of applications help the cleansing process: enemas, liver wraps, breathing exercises, showers, baths, sauna and massages. The Russian doctors recommend in addition two to three hours of light exercise in the open air, like walking. All of this supports the process of detoxification and prompts the functions of kidneys, bowel, liver, lungs and skin. Harmful metabolic products should leave the body and no symptoms of self-poisoning will manifest even during fasts as long as 30 to 40 days.[19]

THE PAST AND HOW IT ALL STARTED

As it was so often the case with big discoveries, it takes a coincidence and a competent researcher to come together.

It all started in the 1950s at the psychiatric clinic of Korsakov in Moscow. It was a time when straitjackets, drugs and force-feeding were a common therapy form for mentally ill people. When psychiatrist Juri Nikolaev met a depressed patient who refused to eat, he decided to trust the sick patient's instinct.

To his own surprise, the psychiatrist noticed from day five onwards the patient opened his eyes and displayed decreased negativism. On day ten he started walking; so far, he had not spoken. On day 15 he drank a glass of apple juice. He went for a walk and gradually re-entered social life. Eventually, the man got well. Who would have thought: a mentally ill patient cured through fasting! Nikolaev did not stop here. The phenomenal success exceeded all expectations and soon he had a waiting list full of people yearning for his therapy. Nikolaev treated patients with schizophrenia, depression, phobia and obsessive-compulsive disorder. Prescribed cures lasted on average 25 to 30 days, and sometimes even up to 40 days.

However, not everyone was convinced of his methods. Russian medical professionals questioned his therapy early on.

They found it difficult to support the unexplored. Hunger was always perceived as an evil, now it is supposed to heal?

Nikolaev started an extensive research project that would silence his critics and re-write the history of science. A number of tests were run on hundreds of patients during and after the fasting cure: physiological and biochemical examinations, determination of hormone levels, encephalograms. A connection between physical change and improved health was observed. Soon the doctors noticed that fasting not only had an impact on psychological deviations and mental disorders but more so on the patients' personality. Dr. Valery Gurvich, one of the psychiatrists who worked in the team of medical professionals for 18 years alongside Nikolaev shared more insights. He observed psychostimulatory and anti-depressive effects in the fasting patients. The effects were evident both, during the first week of fasting and in the refeeding phase. In addition, fasting had a sedative effect which occurred after the fasting crises and could be seen as a turning point for the patient.

Nikolaev treated more than 8,000 patients. Fasting brought about a substantial improvement in over 70% of them, which was still noticeable six years later in 47% of the patients. Some of them were able to lead a regular life and start a family. To the surprise of Nikolaev and his team, not only the mental but also the physical health of his patients improved, in particular eczema, high blood pressure, asthma and polyarthritis. Given the magnitude of the results Nikolaev decided to inform the authorities.

At first skeptical, the General Directorate of Treatment and Preventive Care of the USSR Ministry of Health started a campaign to check the findings in 1973. The National Scientific Research Institute of Pulmonology was tasked to study the therapeutic possibilities, among them were the military doctors Alexey Kokosov and Valery Maximov. They had never heard of fasting cures before and were now in charge of not only proofing the method works but also explaining the reasons. Examined were gastric secretion, the liver, the pancreas and the intestines, as well as gut bacteria, immune status, mineral metabolism and vitamins. Thousands of patients took part in the extensive study. The physicians confirmed Nikolaev's results.[20] Detailed lists with indications and contra-indications were drawn up.[21]

[In medicine the term "indication" is used when a medical treatment is appropriate; "contra-indication" is a condition that serves as a reason to not take a certain medical treatment due to the harm that it could cause the patient.]

Indication	**Contra-indication**
Bronchial disease	Cancer
Cardiovascular disease	Tuberculosis
Gastrointestinal disorders	Diabetes type 1
Endocrine diseases	Chronic hepatitis
Disease of the digestive organs	Thrombophlebitis
Joint and bone disease	Anorexia
Skin disease	Hyperthyroidism

Relative contra-indications include:

- Hypotonic neurocirculatory dystonia;
- Gallstones with highly lithogenic bile;
- Urolithiasis;
- Gastric and duodenal ulcers;
- Phlebeurysm;
- Iron-deficiency anemia;
- Gout;
- Pregnancy and lactation;
- Early childhood (0 – 14) and old age (after 75 years);
- Certain acute respiratory (viral) diseases;
- Persistent cardiac rhythm and conduction disturbances.

Later in the book you will see that prolonged fasting is actually possible for people 75+ years old.

The question remains as to how the effects of fasting can be explained. Fasting causes stress in the organism. This stress leads to self-regulating mechanisms, the sanogenesis, that are normally suppressed. Stress triggers an adaptive response to changed environmental conditions; in this case the deprivation of food. As soon as the organism notices the missing nutrition, it is put on alert. Hormonal and neuroendocrine changes take place and body reserves are mobilized by the hormones; some of which have anti-inflammatory properties.

The Russian physicians were of the opinion that the therapeutic effects were triggered by those self-regulating mechanisms. Various values improved: blood sugar, cholesterol, triglycerides and insulin levels. At the same time, energy expenditure was gradually reduced and breathing, cardiac rhythm and blood pressure were slowing down. Finally, the digestive system was found in a resting state.

Professor Sergeij Osinin, a specialist in bronchial asthma, had more insights on what was happening during prolonged fasts. As a student of Kokosov, the pulmonologist instructed 10,000 asthmatics to fast. No complications were recorded over four decades. One of his studies looked into the cells of the pulmonary lining. In patients with bronchial spasms, these cells will appear black and cause hypersecretion. This indicates the presence of histamine, an amine released when tissue is injured or an allergic and inflammatory reaction takes place. After 12 days of fasting, the histamine had vanished and the cells were filled with lipids. The spasms were gone.[22]

The findings are unique and have never been seen before. Not only were all parameters on the current state of the body analyzed but even local changes have been taken into consideration, like the disappearance of substances causing edema or inflammation. Conventional medicine does not know of a cure for bronchial asthma, a chronic disease that sees patience taking drugs their entire life. These drugs, however, only treat the symptoms temporarily.

Prof. Osinin studied the long-term impact of fasting in a research project with 1,000 participants. The results showed that 50% of patients felt an improvement even after seven years, especially those who maintained a healthy diet after the fast. In some cases, several therapeutic fasts were necessary. Approximately 10 to 15% of patients, though, were completely cured.

Data from all over the Soviet Union was collected with the goal to integrate fasting in the health policy of the government. The academy of sciences confirmed the results and published them in impressive volumes, none of which were ever translated.[23]

2.3 Germany

The next stop brings us to Germany. Germans are no strangers to the concept of fasting. A study conducted in 2020 shows that out of 1,908 respondents 57.8% have already fasted for several times in their life.[24]

BUCHINGER

It comes as no surprise that one of the most renowned fasting institutes has existed here since 1953, Buchinger Heilfasten.

Founded by Dr. Otto Buchinger the clinic enjoys a good reputation abroad with over 2,000 people yearly fasting here. Many suffer from chronic diseases, others come as a preventive measure or to combat high blood pressure, diabetes and obesity.

It all started in 1917 when the physician was struck with severe rheumatoid arthritis. His ability to move was soon so limited, he was confined to a wheelchair which led to his discharge from his duty as an army doctor. The psychological strain and helplessness of Western medicine made him explore alternative therapies. Dr. Buchinger underwent his first fasting cure prescribed by Dr. Riedlin who practiced fasting therapies according to traditional methods with great results. After two fasts the physician had fully recovered. Dr. Buchinger dedicated his life to develop therapeutical methods to use fasting.[25]

Many patients suffering from severe inflammatory rheumatic diseases end-up taking medication for life, amongst these drugs is cortisone. The effects of the drug use are massive but can be reduced with fasting cures, and in some cases even completely stopped.

CHARITÉ – UNIVERSITÄTSMEDIZIN BERLIN

At the biggest university clinic of Europe, the Charité Berlin, therapeutic fasts have a long-standing practice. For over ten years, one floor of the adjacent building is reserved for fasting patients. Many university clinics followed its lead and now also offer medically supervised fasts. Therapeutic fasts are becoming an established part of mainstream medicine.

Prof. Andreas Michalsen, head physician at Charité Berlin, led several scientific studies in relation to fasting. He offers these therapies to patients who suffer from rheumatism, metabolic syndrome or heart disease. Without knowing about the Russian research findings, he studied hormonal changes. These include: adrenalin, noradrenalin, dopamine, leptin, serotonin; all of which have a strong impact on the metabolic process and impact the mood. Similar to the findings of the Russian psychiatrists, Michalsen notes an impact of the elevated happiness hormone serotonin on the fasting patients. Further, he observed a reduced pain sensitivity and increased sensitivity of the insulin receptors.[26]

2.4 Hormones and fasting

The human growth hormone (HGH) has shown to increase by over 300% after only three days of fasting, while after one week the increase amounted to 1,250%.[27] Growth hormone plays an important role in the preservation of bone density and muscle mass, as well as making fat available to use as fuel. This would explain why fasting stimulates HGH's growth and how protein in the muscles can be conserved during long fasts. Secretion of this hormone declines normally with age but will continue to be produced when fasting.

During a fast the stress hormone cortisol declines, while adrenalin increases after 24 hours, reaching its peak of 14% after four days of fasting. Normally adrenalin is released when your life is perceived to be in danger but when you fast smaller amounts are released that help move energy out of your fat and muscle glycogen stores to use as an immediate source of energy. Against common belief, fasting increases metabolism, in particular in prolonged fasts.[28]

The positive impact of fasting can be also observed in men with low testosterone levels due to metabolic syndrome. Insulin downregulates testosterone, the important hormone for male reproduction but also muscle growth.[29]

There are currently no studies available on how fertility in women is affected by prolonged fasts but according to Roman, after a fast a hormonal balance is re-established that primes a woman to conceive a child.

Before I went on my first 10-day fast, I was suffering from terrible period cramps that required me to take pain killers. I would take one ibuprofen pill every month at the beginning of my period. Over the year before my fast, I had to take them every month, before that I had better and worse months, some months requiring drug intervention, some not. My first period after ten days of fasting was all of a sudden pain free. I was very surprised – after all, I am not one to take drugs easily, so for me those ibuprofen pills were "life-savers" in dealing with my excruciating pain every month. I thought to myself that I might be back to a pattern of needing pills every other month. So, I decided to see how I felt next time. The pain, as I experienced it before, never came back. That first fast was in October 2019. Since then, I have not taken medication for period cramps. Last year, when I went back to my second fast with Roman, I asked him if this could be linked to the fast. He thought my magnesium absorption was not functioning properly before and the fast restored the pathways.

2.5 Animals and fasting

A different look at the topic was taken by Yvon Le Maho at the French National Centre for Scientific Research (CNRS) in Strasbourg, France. Since the 1970s the ecophysiologist studied animal populations; among them the emperor penguin in the Galapagos islands. Every year the male emperor penguin fasts for a total of about six months. From the moment he finds his breeding ground, the fast starts. The male hatches the egg for about two months, while he awaits the return of the female. From the time arriving at the breeding grounds to the arrival of the hatched chicken, the male spends on average 115 days fasting. Once the female returns, the mates take turns in feeding and fasting.

Early on Le Maho was fascinated by his observation and wondered how the animals survive. As long as the body is living off its reserves, the protein storage is depleted. Something especially relevant for humans, since the heart muscle can be affected. Once 30 to 50% of the protein storage is emptied, the organism dies. Le Maho and his team measured the percentage of protein stored that the emperor penguin breaks down to understand the limitations of fasting. The result was astonishing. Proteins made up only 4% of the daily energy expenditure during a fast while 96% were covered by fats. So, the organism adapted in a smart manner to use little protein. This observation allows for a split into three fasting phases. In the initial phase, it takes the penguin only a few days to reduce its rapid protein utilization, in contrast to humans whom it takes approximately two weeks. In phase two, protein utilization continues at a low rate, now mainly fat reserves are used. Depending on the fat reserves, this phase can last a long time. In emperor penguins, phase two can last up to 100 days. However, as soon as the body has gone through 80% of its fat reserves, the frugal usage of protein is over and the animal enters the third phase. Now it has to urgently find food before it is too late. Since the penguin has to make its way from the colony, which is often located about 100 km (62 miles) from the sea, to feed, the remaining 20% of lipids are used up for this last trip. This shows that the emperor penguins have a built-in alarm system that alerts them at about 20% of remaining fat reserves to leave the colony to feed, anticipating the depletion of energy reserves with a sufficient margin of safety. Humans seem to lack the alarm system to alert them when cumulative protein depletion becomes critical.

Jean-Patrice Robin, a colleague of Le Maho, led an experiment with rats to see if the three phases of protein usage are similar. The results were comparable. It confirmed that the fundamental adaptation process to fasting is comparable in all animals and humans.[30]

To put this into numbers: a 5'7 adult weighing 153.3 lbs. has approximately 33 lbs. in fat reserves. In good health and with access to water, this suffices for about 40 days.[31]

2.6 Cancer and fasting

We will take a look at the research done in the US in regards to aging, cancer treatments and fasting.

UNIVERSTIY OF SOUTHERN CALIFORNIA – LOS ANGELES, USA

Dr. Valter Longo is a professor of gerontology, the study of aging and age-related diseases, at the University of Southern California in Los Angeles, as well as Director of the Longevity and Cancer Program at the IFOM Institute of Molecular Oncology in Milan, Italy.

Dr. Longo had a hunch that fasting can protect the body from all sorts of harmful substances, amongst them the most toxic one: chemotherapy drugs; or drugs that are used to treat cancer. He took a group of cancerous mice and divided them in two groups. The first group was fed a normal diet, the second one fasted for 49 hours. Subsequently all mice were injected with huge amounts of chemotherapy drugs. The dosage was three to five times higher than comparable amounts allowed in humans. The consequences should have been disastrous. Dr. Longo was travelling when the results reached him. All fasting mice survived; all normally fed mice died. The experiment exceeded any expectations. The experiment was repeated in two more laboratories with the same result.

Video recordings of the two mice groups showed the differences after receiving high doses of chemotherapy drugs clearly. The fasting mice were in best health: they moved normally, their coat was smooth, the tissue undamaged and their cognitive functions seemed to be intact. The normally fed mice, on the other hand, seemed sick and hid in the corners of their cages. Thorough analysis showed that the latter's heart and brain were affected. This news was a bombshell. News outlets everywhere broadcasted the findings: fasting protects from side effects of chemotherapy drugs.

The USC Norris Comprehensive Cancer Center, one of the biggest cancer clinics in the US, immediately started a study on cancer patients. To date, only few participants have been recruited. In a first step it was important to show that fasting was harmless to the health of cancer patients. This revolutionary approach was contrary to official recommendations that foresee an increase in calories and protein.[32]

A success of the experiment would mean that dosages of chemotherapy drugs could be increased without harming the patient.

In 2009, 2015, 2016 and 2018 various clinical trials in small groups of cancer patients (in order of the years ten, 20, 13 and 50 patients) showed similar positive effects of fasting in cancer patients. The 2009 study focused on toxicity and side effects after chemotherapy. It showed that fasting can reduce nausea, vomiting, diarrhea, abdominal pain, and mucositis. The ten patients that fasted before or after chemotherapy barely mentioned any side effect, while almost one of the earlier listed symptoms was reported by five out of six patients who received normal feeding. The four patients that fasted for the entire duration of the chemotherapy reported fewer side effects than those undergoing the same treatment without fasting. Noteworthy is also that no higher number of side effects were reported in fasting patients.[33]

The 2015 study demonstrated reduced DNA damage in patients undergoing fasts. The subjects started their fast 24 hours before chemotherapy and it lasted until 24 hours after. While no significant differences were demonstratable on toxicity induced by chemotherapy in patients fasting or not, reduced DNA damages were shown in fasting patients 30 minutes after therapy administration, signifying a protective role of fasting in these cells. In both groups, lymphocytes had the same DNA damage 30 minutes after therapy administration, however, after seven days, DNA damage remained high only in non-fasting groups. It implies the role fasting plays in promoting DNA recovery after chemotherapy.[34]

The 2016 study looked into fasting timing during chemotherapy. They compared how 24-, 48- and 72-hour fasts impacted the reduction of chemotherapy toxicity. It was observed that fasting was safe and feasible for the patients.

Further, the DNA damage in leucocytes was reduced in subjects who fasted for more than 48 hours.[35]

The 2018 study evaluated the differences in overall survival, quality of life and fatigue improvement in patients on a normal diet versus short-term fasting patients during chemotherapy. Once again it was demonstrated that fasting was safe and well tolerated during chemotherapy. It was demonstratable that fasting reduces fatigue and improves quality of life, specifically in the first eight days after chemotherapy.[36]

It is evident that the big challenge is to re-produce the results from the small cancer patient groups to bigger studies with more variety in tumors. The current research cannot make out if fasting is beneficial to certain tumor types only. What can be confirmed is that fasting can protect the organism against oxidative stress and ageing. Scientists are inclined to also believe that fasting reduces cancer cells' ability to survive and adapt, making them therefore more vulnerable to chemotherapy. At the same time, it seems like normal cells respond well to starvation. Fasting induces a stress response which allows the healthy cell to enter a self-maintenance mode which protects it from the toxic effects of both radiotherapy and chemotherapy.

Nora Quinn, a judge from L.A., did not have the time to wait for the large-scale studies to be conducted when she was diagnosed with breast cancer over a decade ago. She stumbled upon an article on Valter Longo's work in the Los Angeles Times and told her oncologist about it. The physician neither encouraged nor discouraged her but figured there was no harm in trying. Quinn received five chemotherapies. She worried about the side effects, her biggest fear, though, was an impairment of her cognitive abilities. Under the supervision of a medic, Quinn fasted for five days before her first cycle of chemotherapy. She felt good and continued going to work. Before the next two cycles her oncologist advised against fasting. She did not tolerate the chemotherapy well and felt sick. She decided to fast before her last two cycles again and this time felt significantly better. Quinn is convinced that she had fewer side effects when she fasted in comparison to her friends who did not fast. She and nine others took part in a study that confirmed that common side effects like fatigue, feeling of faintness, nausea and headaches were significantly reduced in fasting patients.[37]

A next step would be to look into the effectiveness of the chemotherapy itself – does fasting improve the success of a chemotherapy?

Dr. Longo picked liver, heart and muscle cells to observe the relevant section of the DNA strands. By examining the gene expression, the scientist can see how the information encoded in a gene is used to build protein. At first, the gene expression seemed to be normal but after two days of fasting Dr. Longo observed a radical change. Some genes were now overexpressed, others underexpressed. The genes changed the functioning of the cells and switched to operate in protection mode. A healthy cell knows how to adapt to the lack of glucose and other available nutrients; it had billions of years to learn how to switch to protection mode. So, if fasting protects the healthy cells, how does a cancer cell react? After two days of fasting, the gene expression of the cancer cell was contrary to the healthy one. The cancer cells saw a genetic mutation which made them lose their evolutionary memory and with it the knowledge to protect itself. In an environment that provides only little glucose, the cancer cell is unprotected and shows a higher chemosensitivity.

2.7 Ageing, stem cells and fasting

A study from 2014 showed that prolonged fasts that last between 48 and 120 hours (two to five days) help in down-regulating activities that improve resistance to toxins, as seen beneficial in chemotherapy. The breakdown of white blood cells triggers the renewal of the immune system. At the same time, stem cell numbers not only tremendously increase but have also shown to be more efficient. To achieve such profound changes on a cellular level, it is crucial, though, to fast for more than 24 hours.[38] The switch from glycogen to ketones has to be completed. Stem cells play a crucial role in the body's repair of damaged tissue. Stem cells have the unique ability to develop into any new cell type, like blood, liver or nerve cell or just divide and grow in numbers. Since stem cells reproduce, their effectiveness is tainted by the ageing processes in the body, thus, becoming less effective. In the course of one's life, stem cell numbers decrease, leaving the body more prone to diseases. By fasting for more than 24 hours, you allow your immune system to re-boot by triggering stem-cell renewal, while at the same time rejuvenating your body.

3 The Roman Fessler Method for Weight Loss

This chapter will be dedicated to my eye-opening lessons learned from fasting with Roman Fessler at his *Heilfasteninstitut Fessler* in Losenstein, Austria. During the daily two-hour long seminar sessions, Roman explained step-by-step what to eat and why. He shared his knowledge on overall well-being and weight management success for the long-run. The lessons learned will be substantiated by research and scientific findings. I explained previously how extended fasts have many health benefits, especially with curing and preventing various diseases, but in this chapter, I will explain why I think that Roman's method is probably one of the most effective for long-term weight management. So far, I have completed two 10-day fasts in Losenstein with Roman as my *Heilfastenmeister* (meaning he led the course and the seminars) and followed Roman's recommendation of fasting once a week for 36 hours (in my case, I eat my last meal Sunday night and the next meal consumed is on Tuesday morning). This, in combination with various healthy new habits, helped me not only to lose weight but also to maintain the weight loss.

3.1 About the founder

Roman Fessler was born on May 1, 1959 in Vienna, Austria to parents Hermann and Getrude Fessler. His father made his career as a director at the post office, while his mother was a housewife. He grew up as an only child in the 12th district of Vienna where he attended school. He is currently married to his third wife, Jutta who runs the business with him as well as his two daughters from a previous marriage. At a young age, he felt extreme inner unrest which physically manifested at the ages of 15 and 16; while he was 178 cm (5'10) tall, he weighed 105 kg (231.5 lbs.). With the increased weight, his mental and spiritual problems grew. When he talks about his past in his seminars, this time in his life is often described as a period where he felt stripped of his dignity. All of a sudden, he wasn't referred to as "Roman" anymore but kids would make up cruel, derrogatory slurs – he was reduced to his weight by his peers. Especially, the rejection he experienced by women motivated him to change. By intuition, Roman decided to refuse food intake for ten days. He noticed how much better he felt and adapted the food abstinence to his needs. Later on, he learned there was a well-established term for his "discovery": *fasting cures*.

Roman knew early on in his life that he wanted to be self-employed someday. He started off with a career as a wholesaler, and later completed training to be a merchant; the latter he attributes to his success in all his future business endeavors.

At the age of 21, working full-time as a wholesaler, he used an autodidact approach to teach himself fasting cures. A beautiful side-effect was the maintenance of his new body weight of 74 kg (163 lbs.). In 1989 Roman presented for the first time the knowledge he had gained to a group of interested people in the course of a 10-day seminar. The positive response received turned his passion into his profession.

In 1992, after purchasing and renovating the bed and breakfast for a year in Losenstein, he opened his fasting cure institute. He received the first trade license issued by Austria as a health and diet advisor.

Since then, Roman added to his repertoire: a cook book, production and sale of supplements, healthy food items (e.g., sugar alternatives, soup broths, salts, superfoods etc.), a CD for guided meditation of the 7 Asanas, a cosmetic line (from deodorant to facial creams and body lotions), and since COVID a video and online package for fasts from home, with all relevant information one would normally receive during his seminars.

3.2 The setting

I would like to describe the setting you will find when you come to Losenstein. When I booked my first 10-day fast, I had difficulties understanding what I actually signed up for. Also talking to people who are unfamiliar with the concept, I noticed how many misconceptions there were about a conscious abstinence from food. People seem to think they are paying to be starved and thinking they could do the same thing for free from home.

Losenstein is a small village in the countryside of Upper Austria. The institute is surrounded by nature as far as the eye can see. Mountains, hiking trails, waterfalls and the National Park Kalkalpen are all in close proximity. Every ten days, a new course starts with a different main topic: nutrition, spine, anti-aging, cell regeneration, health, hiking and yoga/anti-cellulite and energy refuel. The package includes:

Room for 9 nights	**Variety of organic herbal teas for different needs** (relaxation, sleep, wake-up, stomach ache, draining, improvement of blood pressure and circulation etc.)
Supplements (essential amino acids to maintain muscle mass, fibers for cleansing the gut, good digestion and keeping you full, vitamins, trace minerals)	**3 "meals" per day:** nutritional drink in the morning, fruit puree, vegetable soup or natural yoghurt for lunch and dinner
Exercise program in the morning depending on the main topic	**Seminars** on the main topic of the fast (every day 2 hours packed with knowledge and the latest research)
Guided hiking tours and excursions in the afternoon	**Evening program** (meditation, autogenic training, tarot, seminars etc.)

The reason prolonged fasts are now possible for people 75 years and older lies in the provision of supplements – in particular the supplemented protein. Before the age of supplements, older people were advised against prolonged fasts due to the potential breakdown of the heart muscle. Luckily, older patients who probably benefit the most from fasting can now participate safely.

On the first and last day of the fast your weight and body fat percentage are measured. Participants who have medical concerns can consult with a doctor who is on-site the first day and can be reached throughout the fast.

An important aspect that helps during the retreat, is that everyone in the house is fasting, meaning you will not be exposed to delicious smelling foods. The group setting makes it easier to stay on goal by being surrounded with like-minded folks. You can share struggles and exchange experiences. The fast can be used as an encouragement for a new start. Guests can choose this time as a new start to, for example, abstain from everyday vices like smoking, drinking coffee, energy drinks, alcohol, sodas etc. Roman asks of every smoker who wishes to keep the habit, to refrain from asking other smokers to join them. The rationale behind it is that an addict, will always agree to join and, thus, be tempted to smoke. Access to a chemical-free bathing pond and spa top off the stay. In addition, massages and other therapeutical treatments can be booked.

Lesson 1

Why 10 days of fasting (and not shorter)

One of the first things that confused me when researching fasting offers, were the different durations of fasts offered. From two or three to ten and more days were presented. My immediate preference was a shorter fast of maybe five days – a duration I could easily fit with work, annual leave days and other vacations planned. This seemed to be an expedited, quick cure for my weight issues, without having to sacrifice too much or commit for too long. As I explained in my introduction, Robert, my friend from whom I heard about extended fasts for the first time insisted that a fast had to last ten days; and now I know why. Studies showed that shorter fasting periods might lead to re-poisoning. This can happen from day five to seven. The reason being that from day four onwards, the toxins are temporarily stored in the lymphatics for one to two days. Up until day nine more and more toxins are stored in the lymph gland. Only then the body starts eliminating toxins, thus, the recommendation to break the fast from day eleven.[39] The other reason has to do with the set-point which will be explained in lesson three.

Lesson 2

Why diets don't work

Diets in this context refer to calorie reduction over a limited period of time.

Most of us will have learned that if you consume less calories than you burn, you will lose weight. So, all you have to do is reduce your caloric intake, maintain your caloric expenditure and over time you will lose weight, correct? Not quite. What actually happens is that with the decrease in calories in, a decrease in calories out is triggered. A study in 1919 showed that a 30% reduction in caloric intake led to a 30% decrease in caloric expenditure. In the end, minimal weight loss was achieved. Your body is an expert in preserving energy. Once it notices the lack of calories, it adapts all systems to run on less fuel. Physiologically this will be evident in a slower heart rate, decreased heart stroke volume and blood pressure, as well as a drop in your body temperature.

People obsess over calories in when the caloric expenditure is often neglected. Exercise is often perceived as the main way of energy leaving the body but little thought is put into the accumulative effect of the below factors, also known as the total energy expenditure:

Basal metabolic rate (calories you burn maintaing body functions at rest)

Thermogenic effects

- Thermogenesis from non-exercise activity (energy expended for everything done that is not sleeping, eating or sports-like exercising, like fidgeting, gardening, shopping, houshold work etc.)
- Diet induced thermogenesis (energy used for digestion and absorption of food)

Exercise

- Excess post-exercise oxygen consumption (also known as the afterburn; energy used in cellular repair, replenishment of fuel stores, recovery activites after exercise)

As much as you wish to control where the calories in go in your body, it is your organism that assesses whether fuel is used for heat, bone and muscle production, digestion, detoxification *or* storage of fat.[40]

This was most evidently demonstrated in The Minnesota Starvation Experiment conducted in 1944 and 1945. The war had left a food deprived, starving population. Scientists had little knowledge on how to refeed humans and wanted to scientifically find the most effective way. The experiment shed new light on the physiological and psychological effects of semistarvation. It subjected 36 healthy participants to a regiment of semistarvation followed by a refeeding phase. The following feeding schedule was set:

Duration	**Calories**
3 months	3,200 kcal
6 months semistarvation	1,800 kcal
3 months nutritional rehabilitation period	Randomly assigned to 1 of 4 energy intake groups (around 2,000 kcal)

The participants continued with work and studies but were expected to walk 22 miles (35.4 km) per week and expend 3009 calories per day. Throughout the experiment physical functions were measured and observed. A personality test and the psychological state of each participant were recorded.

One of the set goals was for participants to achieve a weight reduction of 25% or approximately 2.5 lbs. (1.1 kg) per week by the end of the six months of semistarvation. Food portions depended on the weekly weight loss goal and were accordingly adjusted every seven days.

Over the course of the six months, the participants noticed the following changes:

Extreme tiredness	Muscle soreness
Decreased tolerance for cold temperatures	Dizziness
Decreased energy levels	Food obsession
Increased irritability	Increased impatience
Loss of sex drive	Edema

32 of the 36 initial study objects completed the experiment. It took participants from two months up to two years to feel like they had fully recovered with none of the men feeling "normal"

after the three months of refeeding. Constant hunger was another condition. They constantly overate, to the point where they felt physically sick.

The following physiological changes were recorded:

Resting metabolic rate dropped by 40%	Strength decreased by 21%
Body temperature dropped to an average of 95.8°F (typical adult's is between 97 and 99°F)	Physical endurance dropped by 50%
Blood pressure dropped	Heart rate slowed from an average of 55 beats per minute to 35 bpm
Brittle nails	Hair loss

The body does not know that the calorie restriction lasts only a couple months. It immediately turns down energy expenditure. Instead of losing an average of 78 pounds (35.3 kg), the men lost less than 50%, only 37 pounds (16.8 kg). Their body adapted from using 3,000 calories per day to around 1,800 calories. Their weight loss slowed down.[41]

The only problem is that once the body settles at a lower metabolic base rate from reduced calories in, it stays there for a very long time. This was impressively demonstrated in another study conducted in 2008. The study showed that the subjects that had lost more than 10 % of body weight and were able to maintain that loss for over a year, had reduced energy expenditure levels which persisted well beyond the time of actively trying to lose weight. Data shows that the systems responsible for regulating energy intake and output after weight loss, when in maintenance mode, favor a regain of the lost weight. Further, leptin, the hormone that controls appetite by signaling you when to stop eating, seems to return to its levels from before the weight loss, thus, reversing many of the changes.[42]

A scientific paper from 2011 seems to confirm these results. Weight loss leads to a significant reduction in leptin and increase in ghrelin, the hunger hormone signaling your body to eat. At the same time, satiation from meals decreased. Satiety hormones, amylin, peptide YY and cholecystokinin, are suppressed.[43]

Let's put this into numbers. As an example, we will take a man with an initial caloric intake of 2,800 calories. At 2,800 calories he maintains his weight. He decides to go on a diet of 2,200 calories. The body will adapt all its functions by reducing the expenditure side. At first, he will lose weight successfully and quickly but after a while it stagnates. At the same time, his hormones will signal him to eat the pre-diet calories. His frustration grows, he cannot lose more weight and eventually he will give up the diet. He starts eating "normally" again. However, his body is still set to sustain itself at 2,200 calories. Eating now 2,800 and more calories, he puts back on all the weight and even a little more than before the diet. We can even assume that he is happy with the weight loss and now decides to consciously end the diet. The result would be the same: the weight would be put back on. The decrease in energy intake from food triggers an almost immediate slow-down of the metabolism which persists more or less indefinitely.

So, if diets don't work, what does? This brings me to the next major lesson learned. The Set-point.

Lesson 3

The Set-point

The Set-point theory assumes that homeostatic mechanisms in your body defend a pre-set weight baseline against changes, both up and down. If you lose weight, compensatory mechanisms are triggered to increase it; if you gain weight, the same mechanisms will try to lower it.[44] With obesity, the problem is that this set-point is too high.

The Set-point does not increase with fat, only with sugar and carbohydrates when excess amounts of insulin are released. The Set-point can be lastingly lowered when insulin levels are kept consistently low for ten days or when exercise and proper nutrition are maintained over a long period of time. After that, it is crucial to strictly follow the re-feeding phase in which calories are gradually increased and your stomach resumes its functions step-by-step.[45]

Roman couldn't stress enough that the goal after the 10-day fast and the re-feeding phase should be to maintain the new Set-point until the next extended fast. The goal should not be to lose more weight by reducing calories. The first couple months most people find it easy to maintain the new weight. All the lectures are fresh in your mind, you are motived by your new body and the admiration from your peers. However, after approximately six months, your body will try to creep up to its original weight. You will allow yourself a piece of cake here and a pizza with friends there. The mandatory Thanksgiving and Christmas dinner can of course not be missed. Feel free to list your own feasts and events of the year; the result will be the same – there will be social gatherings that will compromise your diet. Now you might think *"I can make some exceptions, right?"* Wrong. Without any control mechanisms in place, you will regain all your weight. To avoid regaining the weight, Roman recommends a 36-hour fast once per week. Realistically speaking, you will not be able to eat 100% clean for the rest of your days. More benefits of the 36-hour fast will be further elaborated on in the last lesson.

Lesson 4

Insulin resistance and why you shouldn't snack

Insulin resistance is the result of your cells not reacting to insulin anymore. Insulin is needed to move sugar inside the cells. When the process of insulin attaching itself to insulin receptors on a cell to activate enzymes that escort glucose into muscle cells is disrupted, problems arise. In type 1 diabetes, insulin cells produced by the pancreas are destroyed and as a result insufficient insulin is present to escort sugar inside the cells. In type 2 diabetes, however, enough insulin is available but the insulin cannot enter the cell. Sugar left in the bloodstream, causes damage to vital organs over time. So, what happened to our key (insulin) that it can't seem to open the door (cell) anymore? The answer lies in intramyocellular lipids, or in other words the fat inside our muscle cells. Fat that circulates in the bloodstream, irrespective of whether it is from your fat stores or your diet, can have damaging effects when it builds up inside the muscle cell. A build-up of fat in the bloodstream can cause toxic breakdown products that release free radicals which in turn block the insulin-signaling process. Using MRI technology, the impact of high exposure to free fatty acids on insulin resistance can be shown – the increase of fat shows an increase in insulin resistance within 160 minutes. Once fat is reduced from the diet, though, insulin starts working better again.[46]

Dr. Jason Fung impressively explained in his book *"The Obesity Code"* how the food industry and doctors instilled in people to snack and therefore eat several meals throughout the day. One argument was that metabolism is activated after you eat, the so-called thermogenic effect of food. Even though the metabolic rate does slightly increase after a meal, this increase is not significant enough to see actual weight loss. Quite the opposite happens: even though people who would consume a snack, consume slightly fewer calories in the following meal, the reduction is not substantial enough to offset the extra calories of the snack itself. You snack, you eat more, you get fat. More importantly, though, the period of decreased insulin, which translates to fasting, is getting shorter and shorter, while times of increased insulin levels are getting longer. A 30% drop of average time between meals has been recorded between 1977 and 2003, from 271 minutes to 208 minutes. Insulin resistance causes obesity by combining two major factors: over a long period of time, consistently high insulin levels are maintained. If you look back to the 1960s, processed foods rich in refined carbohydrates and sugar were widely available. Less sugar was, however, consumed and obesity was not a major concern. Insulin levels did spike but people at least stuck to three meals a day. Insulin levels could come down between meals and overnight. Nowadays, with all the additional meals throughout the day, these insulin levels don't come down enough and if this persists over a long period of time, obesity and type 2 diabetes are the result.[47]

Lesson 5

Fat cells don't go away with weight loss

The number of fat cells we have is genetically pre-determined and only changes in childhood and adolescence. Once an adult, this number does not decrease, even when weight is lost. Fat cells just shrink in volume but do not disappear.[48] A person with a large number of fat cells early on in life is therefore more prone to becoming obese compared to a lean individual. A fat cell filled to the brim can leak excessive fat into the bloodstream: the consequence are free fatty acids that are not packed into triglycerides and thus, trigger an inflammation.

However, when a person continuously overeats so that fat cells grow too rapidly, it can trigger a reaction in the body which leads to cell division for production of *more* fat cells. These cells, in turn, get fatter faster than normal fat cells. While a lean person has about 25 to 30 billion fat cells, the number for an obese person can be ten times as high, ranging from 250 to 300 billion.[49]

Fat cells also play a vital role in our hormonal balance, mainly in secreting hormones and key signaling molecules for the regulation of metabolism.

These hormones are:[50]

Leptin

- responisble for control and suppresion of appetite

Adiponectin

- increases the body's sensitivity to insulin and aids in the control of blood sugar levels

Estrogen

- stored and produced by fat cells; reason for increased breast cancer risk in overweight people

Angiotensin

- involved in blood pressure regulation

In healthy people, leptin is secreted once they eat enough. Leptin communicates to the brain, the hypothalamus, that enough food has been consumed. The more fat tissue one has, the more leptin is released. Your body naturally tries to prevent you from getting fat. So, what happens in obese people?

Even though leptin is present in obese people, it was found that their brain developed a decreased sensitivity, meaning that the presence of leptin, the hormone signaling that appetite has been satisfied, does not stop these individuals from eating more and subsequently gain weight. As Dr. Fung stated in his book *"The Obesity Code"* 'Obesity is a state of leptin resistance'. Hormonal imbalance of leptin and insulin are key players in the development of obesity.[51]

The lesson here is that your body will always try to re-fill those fat cells, so regular fasts with a healthy lifestyle are the winning combination – not a short-term calorie reduction.

Lesson 6

Brown fat vs white fat – and why you should do cold exposure

Babies are born with brown fat (brown adipose tissue, BAT) that allows them to generate heat and regulate their temperature since they cannot move around when cold. As one grows older, the brown fat decreases and almost disappears in most adults – they are left with white fat. BAT, however, is metabolically active and capable of energy combustion due to containing way more mitochondria than white fat which consists of large droplets of fatty acids. By breaking down glucose and fat, heat is created from BAT. White fat stores excess energy, while brown fat uses glucose and white fat to create energy. As an adult, without any intervention, all you will be left with is white fat. Too much white fat, especially around your organs in the midsection, is confirmed to be a contributing factor to obesity, diabetes and heart disease.

Researchers found that BAT can be activated through cold exposure, like cold showers, ice baths or exposure to temperatures not below 66 degrees Fahrenheit (19 degrees Celsius) for two hours each day (no shivering, though).[52]

Wim Hof, a Dutch extreme athlete with the nickname "The Iceman", has developed a method, called the Wim Hof Method, that combines breathing exercises, cold exposure and cultivation of the mindset resulting in incredible health benefits. At 52 years, he possessed the same amount of brown fat as young adults, showing a metabolization of four and a half times more energy from brown fat.[53] A gene variant in Inuit, the indigenous people inhabiting the Arctic region, for instance, is believed to promote growth of more brown fat as a reaction to extreme cold exposure throughout the year.[54]

Researchers have shown in mice that every-other-day fasting resulted in browning of white fat. It seems like a shift in the gut flora stimulates this metabolic improvement by changing the composition of the microbiome.[55] More on gut flora will follow in lesson 25.

Lesson 7

Trans fats – and why you should avoid margarine and Fast-Food restaurants

Trans fats have become an increasing concern for consumers – and justifiably so!

Before we look into trans fats, let's sort out the differences and health implications of saturated and unsaturated fats. The saturation refers to the chemical structure of the fat. Saturated fats have no double bonds and are saturated with hydrogen atoms. Examples for saturated fats are dairy products like whole milk, cheese, butter, ghee, processed meats like bacon, sausage, salami, fatty cuts of meat, and coconut and palm oil. Saturated fats make oils hard. In general, you can say that the harder the oil, the more saturated fats it probably contains. Unsaturated fats have one or more double bonds and can be further categorized as mono- and polyunsaturated fats. At room temperature they are liquid. Examples include vegetable oils, seeds, nuts, avocados and fish rich in omega-3. Ideally, the consumption of saturated fats should be limited due to them raising low-density lipoprotein (LDL), otherwise also known as bad cholesterol. Unsaturated fats, on the other hand, are said to improve cholesterol levels by increasing high-density lipoproteins (HDL) and reduce blood clots.

Even though, unsaturated fats are generally considered as healthy, trans fats are the exception to the rule. Trans fats are unsaturated fats that increase bad cholesterol, LDL, lower good cholesterol HDL and cause fatty deposits in blood vessels that can lead to heart attacks and strokes. Trans fats clog arteries by sticking to the cell wall, therefore, inhibiting permeability and functions. Trans fats are linked to the increase of fat in the abdominal cavity, insulin resistance and diabetes mellitus type

2. While the body needs fat to function, a better source are unsaturated fats, like nuts, seeds, avocado, peanuts and olives.

Trans fats develop when unsaturated, healthy but liquid vegetable oil is industrially hardened. Through a process called hydrogenation the otherwise liquid vegetable oil can be made solid and given the desired physical properties people normally enjoy in butter by using a catalyst. Nickel is a common catalyst used in commercial hydrogenation of edible oils.[56] Apart from the trans fats that form, the industry has problems getting the nickel out of the end product. Small trace amounts of nickel remain in the oil and are believed to be a contributing factor, with trans fats, to diseases like eczema, hay fever and asthma.

The "International Study of Asthma and Allergies in childhood" is an initiative that started in 1991 and studied in its first phase 721,601 young children and teenagers in 56 countries. The researchers were able to conclude that children that eat fast-food at least three times per week, were associated with a higher risk of asthma, hay fever and eczema. At the same time, three portions of fruit per week seem to counteract these effects.[57]

Another process that leads to the formation of trans fats is the treatment of fats and oils with heat; crucial here is the temperature, duration and how often the same oil is re-heated. Depending on the composition of the fat, and the amount of saturated fats, the temperature affecting a breakdown in the molecular structure can vary.[58] In the food industry this ingredient can be listed as hydrogenated oil or partially hydrogenated oil (PHO). The ingredients label should be carefully studied when "vegetable shortening" is presented: this is a process that was invented in the 90s as a cheap alternative to butter; the problem is that vegetable shortening is typically made from partially hydrogenated vegetable oil. The industry claims that fully hydrogenated vegetable oil has reduced trans-fat amounts in its final product.[59]

Naturally, small amounts of trans fats also occur in meat and dairy products but should only be a concern to people eating diets heavy in full-fat dairy and high-fat meats.

Officially trans fats have been banned by the Food and Drug Administration (FDA) in the US. The process started in 2015, with the FDA's plan to eliminate trans fats from processed foods by giving manufacturers three years initially (but then extended to January 1, 2021) to remove partially hydrogenated oils from their food production. The Centers for Disease Control and Prevention (CDC) estimated that around 20,000 heart attacks each year could be prevented this way.[60] However, if a food product contains less than 0.5 g of trans fat in a serving, it is *required* to declare the product as 0 g trans fat. On the FDA's website, further is explained *"In the absence of these claims, the statement 'Not a significant source of trans fat' may be placed at the bottom of the table of nutrient values in lieu of declaring '0 g' of trans fat".*[61] Eating large amounts or several servings will not prevent trans fat consumption. Especially, when you think of some suggested serving sizes, like in Ketchup, where it is 1 tablespoon (or 3 teaspoons), you will realize soon that suggested portion sizes are often far from the amounts devoured.

Foods rich in trans fats are fried and ready meals such as fries, frozen pizza and burgers, as well as croissants, cookies, chips and microwave popcorn. Next time you want to order fries from a fast-food joint, just consider that the frying oil has been probably used more than once.

It is recommended to use oils and fats with a high smoke point for frying and cooking, such as ghee, clarified butter, coconut oil, as well as corn, sunflower, peanut, soja and canola oil. Butter should not turn brown and oils should not start smoking otherwise that is a sign of oxidation and the product is harmful to your health. Cold-pressed oils and oils made of wheatgerm are not suitable for cooking. Most importantly though, oils should never be reused.

Lesson 8

Cholesterol and the pharma industry

The way cholesterol is measured is in milligrams per deciliter of blood (mg/dL) by looking at the low-density lipoprotein, or LDL, the high-density lipoprotein, or HDL, your triglycerides, or blood fats, and the total cholesterol. To help you remember the different cholesterol types, try to think of **L**DL as the **l**ousy one and **H**DL as the one that makes you **h**appy.

LDL at around 70 mg/dL corresponds to a total cholesterol reading of approximately 150; a level below which no deaths from coronary heart disease are recorded. In the United States, however, the average level hangs around 200 mg/dL.[62] Over the years, doctors started to prescribe cholesterol lowering medication at lower and lower levels. What started almost 60 years ago as a prescription at levels over 260 mg/dL, was gradually reduced to 240, then 220 and now lingers at around 200.[63] Conveniently, more and more patients could be prescribed cholesterol-lowering drugs, also known as statins, that they have to take until the end of their days, thereby making statins one of the best sellers in medicine. Patients with cardiovascular problems, diabetes or high-risk factors of a stroke or heart attack benefit from statin therapy and might accept the risk of potential side effects; for all others due consideration should be given before committing to these drugs.

Let's take a look at what the problem with cholesterol is all about. The build-up of plaque in arteries causes arteriosclerosis which promotes heart disease. While dietary cholesterol is often perceived as the main cause of heart disease, current research implies that plaque, in fact, develops as a response to injury of the artery wall. When the walls become damaged, an inflammatory reaction is triggered which allows for the cholesterol to penetrate the artery wall, build up plaque and cause proliferation of smooth muscle. A rupture in plaque is essentially what leads to a heart attack: the rupture causes a blood clot which blocks the artery, resulting in a lack of oxygen. This would explain why heart attacks and strokes can be classified as inflammatory diseases, rather than simply blaming cholesterol levels.[64, 65] Cholesterol is for that matter a crucial building block in the membranes surrounding all cells and also needed to make bile salts which are required to break down fat in the body. People low in cholesterol often have problems digesting fats. If you do not get enough cholesterol through your diet, the liver will manufacture it. In fact, 80% of cholesterol is made by the liver and only 20% are consumed through diet.[66]

Breast cancer cells feed on LDL cholesterol, allowing them to promote their own growth. The cancer is believed to use the cholesterol to produce estrogen. Further, the bad cholesterol can support tumor membranes and thus, help the cancer spread into more tissues. Now, this could make one wonder, if statins are maybe useful in the prevention of breast cancer. After all, the lack of LDL cholesterol, should hinder the growth of invasive breast cancer. However, a study conducted in 2013 of thousands of women with breast cancer reported using statins for a decade or longer can lead to double the risk of invasive breast cancer in postmenopausal women.[67] Other side effects of statins include memory loss, confusion, liver and muscle damage, as well as kidney failure and offset of diabetes 2 by increasing insulin resistance.

Fasting in combination with a healthy diet is a safe way of not only stopping progress of coronary diseases but actually reversing them – without harmful side effects! Like with all inflammatory diseases, the abstinence of food lowers inflammations in the body. Vegetables, like kale, administered in large quantities have shown to lower LDL and boost HDL within three months due to the increase of antioxidant activity in the blood.

Lesson 9

Fatty liver – and why you don't need breakfast

On a day-to-day basis, the body uses glucose for energy. The excess glucose that is not needed immediately is saved as glycogen in the liver. If you constantly overeat, more glycogen is saved around your liver as fat – you develop a fatty liver. A major contributor to a fatty liver in obese individuals, is fructose and its metabolization in the body. Commonly fructose was consumed in small amounts as a component of fruits, grains, nuts, seeds and vegetables. In fact, this combination of fructose with fiber and fat is what helps the body with absorption of valuable nutrients.[68]

Looking at the qualities of fructose, what stands out is it being sweeter than glucose and not raising blood glucose significantly. The modern food industry managed to extract fructose from corn and use it as a sugar substitute, also known as high fructose corn syrup. This led to a tremendous increase in fructose consumption. A single glass of juice at times contains the same amount of fructose found in four to five apples. While glucose with the help of insulin can be used as fuel in every cell, fructose can be only metabolized in the liver. Fructose is metabolized further into glucose, lactose and glycogen. The glycogen storage space is limited, however, and once its capacity is exhausted, excess glucose is stored as fat. The process it triggers is called *de novo lipogenesis* and refers to the liver manufacturing fat from glucose. All of a sudden, the liver doesn't get to use up these reserves anymore; quite the opposite happens and it has to shove more and more fat in the already cramped space. For that purpose, it releases more insulin to help with the job but there is simply no space left, leaving the liver insensitive to the efforts of insulin. Were insulin levels to drop suddenly, all the fat and sugar would be pouring back into the bloodstream, therefore insulin levels have to remain high. The vicious cycle is set: insulin resistance leads to higher insulin levels.[69]

In 1980 healthy individuals were given an extra 1,000 calories per day of either fructose or glucose. In only seven days, the fructose group had a 25% worse insulin sensitivity, while the glucose group reported no change in insulin sensitivity.[70] In 2009 a study showed how pre-diabetes can be induced in as little as eight weeks by feeding healthy subjects 25% of their daily calories as Kool-Aid sweetened with fructose. The group consuming the same amounts of the sweet drink with glucose did not show such high insulin levels and insulin resistance.[71]

In order to allow these reserves to be depleted, Roman suggests to not eat for the first two to three hours after you wake up, mainly because your body does not need energy from food at this point. Now there will be two groups of people: one group confirming that they actually aren't hungry right after they get up but due to some advice they found online, claiming that breakfast is the most important meal, they force themselves to breakfast. The other group will claim they absolutely need food first thing in the morning, otherwise they cannot function, they feel weak and faint without food in the morning. They will claim their blood sugar is just too low that early in the day and they get headaches. It is possible, though, to start your day without eating right away in the morning! Our bodies are set out to endure dips in blood sugar levels. In fact, our bodies produce a cocktail of hormones that fuel us up without actually needing an external source. This effect is called the dawn phenomenon and happens every morning before we wake up. A combination of growth hormone, cortisol, epinephrine and norepinephrine (adrenalin) is released into our bodies and triggers the liver to produce new glucose. While it is believed that by eating a large breakfast (the meal that actually breaks your fast), less calories are consumed the rest of the day, science shows that lunch and dinner portions seem to not decrease in calories, irrespective of the calories consumed at breakfast. Even worse so, breakfast eaters seem to eat more and more often as a study in 2014 showed. The study looked into breakfast habits of normal and overweight people and assessed changes to nutrient and energy intake consumption patterns. A popular belief was also that breakfast aids your metabolism. This was not found to be true in a study in England where subjects in a randomized controlled trial aged 21 to 60 were observed for three years. Total energy expenditure remained the same, whether breakfast was eaten or not. However, breakfast eaters consumed an average of 539 calories more per day compared to those skipping breakfast.[72]

A liver that is constantly inflated with fat, always inflamed and never gets a break is prone to illness. A fatty liver left untreated can develop scarring which eventually will cause liver failure. Excessive alcohol consumption is the other major cause for accumulation of fat in the liver. Liver cirrhosis is commonly associated with scarring caused by heavy drinking over a long period of time but can, in fact, also hit people as a result of their diet which is then referred to as nonalcoholic fatty liver disease. The best example of how rapidly a bad diet can affect your liver was given in the documentary "Super Size Me". For a month, Morgan Spurlock ate exclusively McDonald's with the result of more weight, higher blood pressure and cholesterol, and elevated levels of liver enzymes. The latter is a sign of liver cells dying and leaking their contents into the bloodstream. A group of Swedish researchers tried to replicate the documentary's findings by making a group of people eat fast food twice a day. After only seven days on this diet, the formerly normal liver enzyme levels were elevated by more than 75%.

Whole grains, like oatmeal, whole grain rice and whole grain bread, are found to decrease the risk of liver inflammation. Cranberries were found to suppress most effectively the growth of human liver cancer cells, probably due to a plant compound called anthocyanins. The purple, red, and blue pigments in such fruits and vegetables as berries, currants, grapes, plums, red cabbage, purple sweet potato, kidney beans, tomatoes and red onion, were shown to prevent fat accumulation in human liver cells in in vitro studies.[73] Do your liver, and yourselves, a favor and skip breakfast!

Lesson 10

Blood sugar levels and why you are hungry the morning after an all-you-can-eat buffet

Let's say you eat a good source of complex carbohydrates like beans. Your blood sugar will gradually rise after your meal, insulin is slowly released and after a while your blood sugar levels will gradually drop again to the natural lower end. You experience fullness for a long time and do not "crash" after your meal.

Now let's look at what happens when you eat a meal rich in simple carbohydrates, like sugar or complex carbohydrates like bread. Bread, against common believe, is a complex carbohydrate but raises blood sugar levels significantly with a barely noticeable difference between white and whole grain bread. These carbohydrates are easily broken down in the body. In a short amount of time large amounts of insulin are released. The blood sugar level spikes. The consequence is an equally quick drop. The only problem is that after such an excessive rise the blood sugar doesn't just drop to the fasting level but it tumbles so far down that a glucose crash is caused, a so-called insulin-induced hypoglycemia. Symptoms include hunger and the craving for sugar and carbohydrate-rich foods – a quick fix. The vicious circle starts: you overeat, crash, eat more sugary foods, crash. People will experience crashes after big, unbalanced meals feeling tired and exhausted. The same mechanisms come into play after indulging in an all-you-can-eat buffet the night before. If you have experienced this before, you know the feeling of hunger the next morning. You had just eaten well beyond your body's needs but wake up 12 hours later feeling hungrier than ever – how is that possible? The sharp increase in blood sugar, followed by the blood sugar dropping below your body's fasting level is the culprit. Since your liver stores energy, though, there is no need to eat right away. Give your body time to use that glycogen reserve. Blood sugar is regulated by the hormone insulin. Insulin, in turn, has a major impact on the weight, as you will learn in the next lesson.

Lesson 11

High Insulin = High Weight
Low Insulin = Low Weight
No Insulin = Set point is lowered

The three major lessons are in the headline. High insulin levels are the reason for high weight, low insulin in turn leads to low weight and no insulin (or very little insulin) over a longer period of time brings the set-point down.

The body's set-point is regulated by the amount of insulin in the blood. It is proven that fasting insulin levels in obese people are higher than in lean ones. In addition, the response to food is exaggerated in obese individuals, meaning insulin levels rise much higher in an obese person, than a lean one when the same food is consumed. Over time, high levels of insulin cause weight gain by increasing the set-point.

To prove the first statement, long-term studies were conducted with individuals suffering from type 2 diabetes. Different quantities of insulin were administrated; in one group insulin was directly injected while in the other group a drug was given that increases the body's secretion of insulin. The direct insulin injections, however, raised serum levels more significantly. The shocking result was that both groups gained weight, although the insulin injections caused a bigger weight gain of 9 lbs. (4 kg) in contrast to 6.8 lbs., (3.1 kg) in the group given the drug. The more insulin in your body, the greater is the weight gain.

Even more impressive was the result of a study conducted in 1993 were type 2 diabetis patients were administared high dosages of insulin over the course of six months in combination with a calorie restriction of approximately 300 calories per day. One would assume that calorie reduction has to lead to weight loss, right? Unfortunatley, reducing calories while insulin levels remain high, does not lead to weight loss. Even though the blood sugar levels normalized, all patients gained weight, by an average of 19 lbs. (8.7 kg)! Insulin is the reason for obesity. It is the hormonal imbalance that causes people to gain excessive weight.[74]

Many drugs available nowadays to help type 2 diabetis patients get their high blood sugar levels under control, lead to higher insulin levels which in turn make patients gain even more weight.

On a 10-day fast, the average weight that is lost is about 5 kg (11 lbs.) for women, and 10 kg (22 lbs.) for men. Roman recounted the story of one male guest who had brought his own scale to the institute and kept track of his weight. The guest had barely lost any weight several days into the fast and couldn't understand what was going on. Roman was surprised himself; after all, the guest swore to not have eaten anything, except for the meals provided by the staff. So Roman went to investigate himself by looking into the man's trash. He found the wrapping paper of sugar-free hard candies. It all made sense now: even though these candies do not have any calories, the artificial sugar in them, raise insulin levels. No matter how much calories you cut, if your insulin levels stay up, you cannot lose weight.

Type 2 diabetis patients participating in a therapeutic, prolonged fast stop taking their medication after a couple days because their insulin levels finally drop low enough. After a fast, your insulin sensitivity is high, meaning your body only needs secretion of little insulin to move sugar out of your blood stream. Giving your body breaks between meals, not snacking, and fasting allows those insulin levels to come down.

Lesson 12

Why you should pay more attention to glycemic load rather than to glycemic index

The glycemic index (GI) shows how carbohydrate-containing foods affect blood glucose levels. It is a good indicator of carbohydrate quality. For that purpose, it looks at portions containing 50g of carbohydrate and observes the impact on blood glucose levels after ingestion. Then it compares it against the reference standard which is glucose with a value of 100. Foods low on the GI scale release glucose more slowly and gradually, while the opposite is the case for foods higher up on the scale. On the official website of the glycemic index https://glycemicindex.com an extensive GI database is available. Since fat and protein on their own barely trigger blood glucose levels, they are not included in the database. Interestingly enough, Roman's recommendation on drinking two teaspoons of apple cider vinegar mixed into half a liter of water before every big meal of carbohydrates can be found confirmed here:[75]

Food Name white bread vinegar	GI Search GI	Serving Size (g) Search Serving Size (g)	Carbs Per Serve (g) Search Carbs Per Serve (g	GL Search GL
White bread eaten with 18 g white vinegar (6% acetic acid)	63	30	15	9
White bread eaten with 23 g white vinegar (6% acetic acid)	73	30	15	11
White bread eaten with 28 g white vinegar (6% acetic acid)	54	30	15	8
White bread eaten with vinegar as vinaigrette	45	30	15	7
White bread, containing 2% vinegar and 2.5% sourdough	79	30	12	9

White bread eaten with 28 g white vinegar (6% acetic acid)	54	30	15	8

Food Name:	White bread eaten with 28 g white vinegar (6% acetic acid)
GI:	54
Food Manufacturer:	
Product Category:	Breads
Country:	Sweden
Serving Size (g):	30
Carbs per serve (g):	15
GL:	8
Reference:	Ostman E. Granfeldt Y, Persson L, Björk I. Vinegar supplementation lowers glucose and insulin responses and increases satiety after a bread meal in healthy subjects. Euro J Clin Nutr 2005, 59: 983-8.

Figure 1: *GI of white bread consumed with vinegar*

White bread (100% wheat flour) + 2% pectin	85	30	13	11

Figure 2: *GI of 100% white bread consumed with 2% pectin*

The information on figure 1 about the GI of white bread eaten with 28 g white vinegar (6% acetic acid) stems from a research paper with the title "Vinegar supplementation lowers glucose and insulin responses and increases satiety after a bread meal in healthy subjects".

However, the carbohydrate content of foods varies: for instance, 100 g of an apple contain 14 g of carbohydrates; the average apple weights approximately 120 g, containing 16 g of carbohydrate. You would have to eat roughly three apples to get the carbohydrate content of 50g, now comparable to the GI scale. Hardly anyone would consume three apples at once. Raw apples have an average GI of 34. By this logic, serving size should be considered which is how the glycemic load comes into play. By multiplying the grams of available carbohydrate in a serving size of the food with the food's glycemic index, and then dividing this by 100 you get a number which represents the glycemic load. The glycemic load compares serving sizes of foods.

In the case of a raw apple the calculation is the following:

16 g x 34 = 504/100 = 5.04 → GL = 5

The glycemic load for a white bread bagel is for example 24, while black beans score a 7 and raw carrots a 1! A trend you will notice is that heavily processed carbohydrates, also referred to as refined carbs, contain high concentrations of carbs and score subsequently high in the index, contrary to unprocessed whole foods. Later in the book I will explain why whole grain still matters. Not all carbs are bad!

Lesson 13

Why you should always eat the whole fruit and vegetable (peel & kernel)

One of the first things Roman talks about is the importance of eating, where possible, the entire fruit with its peel and pit, stone, pyrene or kernel. I briefly mentioned earlier that fructose naturally occurs in small amounts in fruits, vegetables, nuts and seeds and that naturally fructose was consumed as part of a whole food. The fiber and fat content of fruits is stored in the peel and kernel which is essential for the absorption of nutrients and the reason your blood sugar levels will not spike after, for example, eating an entire apple – keep in mind with its peel and pits. Now, this is not always possible. If you think of bananas or pine apples, you will not eat the exterior of the fruit. Roman recommends that all stone fruits are consumed with their core, where this is not possible the fruit should be consumed with three almond-sized nuts in order to allow your blood glucose levels to rise steadily from the consumption of fat. The idea is to compare the volume of three almonds and adapt the ratio. If you eat a smaller seed, like pine seeds, you can eat more than three; with junkier nuts, like the Brazil nut, probably two Brazil nuts will make up for three almonds.

In general, fruits should be bought in their most natural state, meaning modified fruits, like seedless grapes or watermelons should be avoided. Obviously, the shell of a watermelon, for instance, cannot be consumed but Roman highly recommends eating the white inner lining which is full of cellulose and rich in fiber. The skin and pith – the white lining between the fruit and skin – of oranges, which actually tastes bitter, is a natural appetite suppressant and full of fiber. The same logic applies to vegetables: where possible, eat the skin and pit. An example would be pumpkin; you already know that pumpkin seeds taste good but you probably still cut it out before preparing the actual vegetable. Important here is to buy organic produce where no pesticides and toxins were sprayed on the skin.

The importance of consuming the whole fruit and vegetable becomes apparent when looking at studies where supplements where used. Antioxidations play a crucial role in the body to eliminate free radicals which cause ageing and damage to the cells. Fruits and vegetable naturally contain high levels of antioxidants. Researchers gave study subjects antioxidant supplements instead of advising them to eat more fruits to treat respiratory or allergic diseases with the result that no beneficial effects were observed. Hundreds of antioxidants work together, creating a synergistical network to help your body get rid of free radicals. Isolated or extracted components in the form of a pill do not have the same effect as eating whole foods. An intake of one antioxidant in high amounts can destabilize this delicate balance and thus, diminish the body's ability to fight diseases.[76,77]

A similar experiment confirmed the importance of eating whole foods versus extracted supplements: women consuming a diet rich in nuts, and thus, rich in vitamin E had almost half the risk of asthma compared to women taking vitamin E supplements, that saw no benefits at all.[78]

Food is not the only trigger for release of insulin. In the next lesson, we will look at the role stress plays in weight management.

Lesson 14

Why stress makes you fat

The psychological state of stress is, in fact, a result of the hormone cortisol being released. From an evolutionary standpoint, short-term stress was common when confronted with a life-or-death situation, or circumstances where a decision had to be made on fight or flight. Physiologically, the release of cortisol means glucose is made available for muscle use, either to fight for your life or to flee – both physically strenuous activities. Nowadays people find themselves in long-term stress situations that range from relationships, work problems, and sleep deprivation. These situations do not require a physical action to survive. Nonetheless, the body physically reacts in the same way: stored energy is made available; blood glucose levels rise. Since this extra glucose is not used by the muscles, insulin is released to lower the blood sugar again.

Research has demonstrated that cortisol injections over a long period of time increased insulin. Even back in 1983, scientists were able to show that treatment of healthy patients with prednisone, the synthetic cortisol, increased glucose levels by 6.5% and insulin levels by 20%. The result always remains the same: a persistent increase in insulin leads to weight gain.

Particularly shocking in this context is the tremendous impact sleep deprivation has on hormone balance. One night of insufficient sleep is enough to increase cortisol levels by more than 100%. Cortisol levels remain elevated by 37% to 45% the next evening. In addition to the decline of insulin sensitivity, leptin and ghrelin, the appetite and hunger hormone, are disrupted.[79]

Reducing stress is vital and can be aided by meditation, yoga or exercise. Something passive, like watching TV or playing video games is not very effective in stress relief. Needless to say, the long-term goal should be to resolve the issues causing stress.

Lesson 15

Carbs – and why whole grain matters

Let's take a look at what makes a grain whole and the implications on your health. While a whole grain contains the bran, that is rich in fiber, and the germ, which contains the fat and vitamins, white bread has the bran and germ removed – the two components helping the body extract valuable nutrients. You are left with an empty endosperm, a concentration of starchy carbohydrates. Visually they differentiate in their color: whole grain bread and pasta is naturally brown. When bran and germ are removed, the color is white. Not even products that read "100% whole grain" have necessarily whole grains in them. 100% wheat, multigrain, stone-ground, cracked wheat, bran or seven-grain are *not* whole grain products. The industry started selling "enriched" white bread, claiming that the natural minerals and nutrients that have been initially removed during milling are put back into the product. However, the lost fiber cannot be retrospectively replaced. The food industry started to sell brown spelt and rye products, confusing some not-so-savvy shoppers, by mixing coffee grounds or raisin juice concentrate into white bread making consumers think they are buying healthy, dark bread.[80]

The main reason you want to consume whole grain products, is for its fiber content. One way to ensure fiber consumption from whole grains, is by following the Five-to-One Rule for packaged goods by Dr. Michael Greger. For every five grams of carbohydrates you eat, you should get one gram of fiber. The idea is to not eat a ton of carbohydrates without getting any fiber. For that purpose, you divide the number of carbohydrates per serving with its fiber content; the number should be smaller or equal to 5. Let's take Canyon Bakehouse Ancient Grain Gluten Free Bread, 100% Whole Grain Sandwich Bread as an example.

Even though, the bread name has "100% whole grain" in the title, the carbohydrate content per serving is 13 g with a fiber content of only 1 g; 13/1 = 13. You'd have to consume 13 g of carbohydrates to get 1 g of fiber; the product does not pass the test – neither does the American classic Wonder 100% Whole Wheat Sliced Bread. With 11 g of carbohydrates to 2 g of fiber, you get a score of 5.5. Ezekiel bread, on the other hand gives you 3 g of fiber per 15 grams of consumed carbohydrates; 15/3 = 5.

Even though, you will read that something is whole wheat, the form you digest it in, makes a difference to your body. A milled grain is absorbed faster which is why your blood sugar will rise quicker after ingesting any sort of flour; as a result, fewer food is left for your friendly gut flora. Eating intact grains versus pureed or grinded grains makes a difference for your body also when it comes to the bulk of stool. Stool significantly increases in size when for example whole chickpeas are ingested (not so much from eating hummus) because of the increased good bacteria growth. You read correctly, it is not the actual food making your stool bulkier but in fact trillions of good bacteria that were able to grow because you ate well![81]

Three portions of whole-grain foods per day showed significant improvements after 12 weeks in a study conducted in middle-aged people in 2010. The study showed how those three portions of whole-grain foods lowered the cardiovascular disease risk through blood pressure lowering mechanisms. Subsequently, the reduction in blood pressure decreases the prevalence of coronary artery disease by 15% and stroke risk by 25%.[82]

People who eat the most whole grains were shown to drastically slowing the narrowing of the two major arteries in the body, the coronary arteries to and from the heart, and the carotid arteries feeding the brain.[83]

Roman's recommendation for whole grain pasta is 70 grams (2.5 ounces) per portion. The pasta should be cooked "al dente", meaning not too soft. This way the pasta will expand further in your stomach, making you full sooner for a longer period of time. Further, its glycemic index is lower compared to overcooked pasta. After eyeballing my pasta sizes for all these years, I couldn't believe how tiny the portion was (especially uncooked)! Over time, 70 grams became more than enough. I started to add vegetables and a protein to my pasta or made a big bowl of salad – and voila! I get to eat pasta in moderation and still feel satiated after my meal.

Another valuable tip Roman gave was to not overcook potatoes. In general, potatoes have many valuable nutrients, many of which can be found in the peel. The heat can not only kill these nutrients but also turn the starch into pure sugar. It is recommended to cook it firm-to-the bite.

Lesson 16

A lesson on protein

The body needs 20 different amino acids, the building blocks of proteins, to perform its functions. Out of these 20 amino acids, nine are essential, meaning they cannot be synthesized by the body, unlike carbohydrates and fat, and thus, must be consumed through one's diet. Animal protein, soy, quinoa, pistachios and buckwheat are the only nutrients that contain all nine essential amino acids.

Tofu is an especially dense source for protein. For a while, soy was believed to increase estrogen and potentially cause health risks. It most probably stems from soy containing phyto*estrogens*, a plant-based compound that mimics estrogen in the body. Too much estrogen is linked to the potential development of breast cancer; at the same time the female sex hormone is essential to bone health. Ideally you want estrogen to display only its positive effects on certain tissues. Here comes soy into play: as some kind of double-agent, it possesses the ability to lower breast cancer risk, an anti-estrogenic effect, while also help reduce menopausal hot-flash symptoms, a pro-estrogenic effect. Many remarkable studies attest to the positive effects of soy phytoestrogens when it comes to both prevention of breast cancer and survival chance once breast cancer has been diagnosed. Other food items rich in phytoestrogens are edamame, flaxseeds, pumpkin seeds, berries, grapes and peanuts.[84]

Common recommendations for daily protein consumption state 0.8 g per kilogram of body weight (0.03 ounces per 2.2 lbs.). Depending on sex, age and activity level this may vary. Below you can find protein content for 100 grams (3.5 ounces) of various foods:

100 G/ 3.5 OZ	PROTEIN CONTENT
TOFU	8 g / 0.3 oz
RED MEAT (RAW)	20 – 24 g / 0.7 – 0.85 oz
QUINOA (RAW)	15 g / 0.5 oz
RED LENTIL (RAW)	24 g / 0.85 oz
CHEDDAR CHEESE	25 g / 0.88 oz

Before I get into some of the studies available, let us look at how many of these studies are conducted. The studies that are available on animal protein are association studies, meaning that certain assumptions are made based on associating factors with each other; findings are not causally determined. For instance, often times people that eat meat, also tend to drink more alcohol or smoke. Some observations might stem from a person eating animal protein, others might be the cumulative effect of eating meat, drinking alcohol and smoking. This is also the reason coffee had such a bad reputation. Scientists saw that coffee drinkers had a higher mortality rate. Coffee drinkers are often also smokers and once the smokers were removed from the data coffee fared better, later even showing its life-prolonging properties![85]

Meat consumption, for instance, is associated with weight gain. Even if calories are maintained, three extra servings of meat per day are associated with one extra pound of weight over one year. Protein from dairy fair better in association studies, claiming that even though insulin levels increase significantly, people eating a lot of whole milk (not low-fat milk though), sour milk, cheese and butter gain less weight. The highest intake of dairy was associated with the lowest incident of developing insulin resistance syndrome like obesity, hypertension and type-2 diabetes.[86] Animal protein is more acid forming due to its high content of sulfur-containing amino acids. Fruits and vegetables, on the other hand, are more base forming and help neutralize acids. Protein that is consumed in excess is converted into sugar and uric acid in the body; excess sugar is stored as fat; the uric acid is stored in the joints. Gout is one example where consumption of too much red meat, organ meats, like liver and kidney, fish that contain large amounts of purines, like shellfish, tuna, anchovies, and sardines or alcoholic beverages, in particular beer and sugary drinks can lead to painful, sudden pain attacks, swelling and tenderness in joints.

When Dr. Campbell was assigned to a nationwide project in the Philippines to look into malnourished children with an unusually high prevalence of liver cancer, a disease commonly only seen in adults, he made an interesting and for him career-defining discovery. At first, the researchers thought that the malnutrition was caused by aflatoxin, one of the most potent carcinogen discovered, which is produced by mold.

At this point it might be worth explaining how cancer even comes to existence. Cancer advances in three stages: initiation, promotion and progression. Initiation is when this first cell is turned cancerous. This can happen when exposure to certain chemicals, also known as carcinogens, cause a mutation. By-products of industrial processes are one example of such chemicals but they can also form in nature, even though in much smaller quantities. The permanent alteration of the gene is evident in a damaged nucleus, or the DNA of the cell. The initiation is completed once daughter cells with the altered/mutated DNA are formed. The initiation phase can happen in a very short amount of time, even a couple minutes. In most cases, initiation is irreversible and remains as a potential source of cancer growth. That's where the promotion stage begins. This stage can take many years. A cluster has to form big enough to become detectable. The promotion stage depends on the right conditions, though. Only in certain environments can cancer cells flourish. If the required conditions are not met, these cells remain dormant. Promotion is *reversible*. Dietary factors have an impact on the promotion stage and can act as promoters or anti-promoters to growth of tumors. Breast cancer, for instance, can have its initiation in puberty but only grow detectable after menopause. In order to grow to a lump big enough to be detected by a physician, it can take many years.

The final stage, progression, begins with the invasion of other tissues by wandering off its initial site. That's when doctors speak of metastases.

In the case of the Philippine children aflatoxin was the carcinogen. The malnutrition was believed to stem from a lack of protein, especially animal protein. For ten years, Dr. Campbell conducted research to come to the shocking conclusion that children with the highest animal protein-diets were most likely to develop liver cancer. The researchers were able to show that rats administered with aflatoxin and a diet of 20% protein developed liver cancer, while the group on a 5% protein diet with the same exposure to aflatoxin avoided liver cancer.[87] Dr. Longo, professor of gerontology, who studies aging and age-related diseases, and about whom we have heard previously in the chapter on cancer and fasting, reached similar conclusions. Over 18 years, he studied data of 6,400 people over the age of 50. He found that people between the ages of 50 and 65 years, that consumed about 20% or more of calories from animal protein compared to individuals consuming 10% or less, had a significantly higher mortality risk. The mortality risk was a staggering 74% higher over the observational period of 18 years in the high-animal protein group with a four times higher cancer risk. At the same time, the data seems to point at beneficial effects of eating more protein after approximately 65 years of age which is observed by a lower mortality risk. Longo and his team went even further to see the potential effect of animal protein on cancer promotion. They injected 20,000 breast cancer cells into female mice. All the mice on the diet rich in animal protein developed tumors within 18 days; the protein-reduced group had a tumor incidence of 70%. 20,000 breast cancer cells are an extremely large amount to be exposed to, therefore, 30% of mice not developing cancer just from a dietary intervention is a remarkable result. Longo, just like Campbell, saw no adverse effect of plant protein on mortality when analyzing the data.[88]

To come back to Dr. Campbell's research, he showed in his 27 years of work that dietary protein has the power to turn on and turn off cancer growth – and that by simply changing the amounts consumed! For humans, 10% protein averages approximately 50 to 60 grams per day (1.7 oz to 2.1 oz), which approximately amounts to the recommended 0.8 grams (0.3 oz) per kilogram of body weight for the average 70 kg (154 lbs.) person. The study showed that casein in particular, a protein that makes up approximately 80% of cow's milk, contributed to the development of cancer in all stages. On the contrary, proteins from plants, including wheat and soy, did not promote cancer, irrespective of intake levels. In his book "The China Study" he comprises more than 8,000 statistically significant findings between diseases and dietary factors.[89]

When we look at some of the diet trends that emerged over the last decades, protein developed a good standing against the two other macronutrients carbohydrates and fats. The followers of the Atkins diet were happy when they learned they could eat endless amounts of meat (no distinction between heavily processed or natural meats, from bacon to sausage, ham, pork, beef and chicken, everything is fair game), as long as none of the other macronutrients were touched. Ironically, many of the processed meats contain mainly fat.

We all know that if you aim for muscle growth, you need protein. No wonder the fitness industry created a million-dollar business with protein powders, shakes and bars. Protein is indeed the building material for all cell growth. There is a molecule in our body, the so-called rapamycin or mTor, that assesses availability of nutrition and energy to signal cell growth. This assessment is based – among other factors – on the availability of protein. While as a child, when we are still growing and developing, it is important to have sufficient protein available for growth, the constant over-stimulation of mTor due to diets high in animal protein at an older age, is not beneficial anymore. As we age, damaged building blocks of protein start to accumulate and clump together in the body, as is the case, for instance, with brain cells in Alzheimer patients. The accumulated waste product of growth and protein is what causes cell aging. At this point, what your body actually needs is a break from food to clean itself; that's where fasting and autophagy come into play. In mice, adhering to a diet that is one week low in protein, followed by a week of a protein-rich diet over several cycles showed a visible slow-down of Alzheimer's development. By reducing the protein in the diet of the mice every other week, less harmful cells were accumulated. Once again, these observations were not made in individuals consuming plant protein.[90]

We shall take a look at how consumption of large amounts of animal protein can impact your organs, in particular your kidneys, in the long run. Consumption of animal protein has been linked to chronic kidney disease; a disease that has increased the most over the past generation. First signs of an impaired kidney are leakage of protein into urine. A healthy kidney is retaining protein and vital nutrients, only filtering useless waste and toxins. Saturated fat, trans fat and cholesterol, all abundantly present in animal protein, can damage the sensitive kidney cells over time. A dramatic increase in the workload of kidneys, normally occurring after eating large amounts of animal protein, induces a state of hyperfiltration. While the kidneys can deal with the occasional sudden, large dose of animal protein, the excessive amounts it has to deal with, by being burdened on a daily basis, are not neglectable anymore. This could explain why kidney function declines the older people get. Plant protein, on the other hand, seems to not burden the kidneys. A six-month long clinical trial examined how kidneys process soy protein contrary to dairy protein with the result that plant protein was found to improve renal function (kidney function) of ailing kidneys.[91]

Let's take a look at protein and its effect on insulin and therefore its impact on weight management. Insulin and blood sugar move independently from each other. This is important to understand since the major focus over the last dacades had been on blood sugar levels rising with the assumption that only what makes your blood sugar rise, impacts insulin secretion. That is also the basis of the glycemic index as it soley looks at the impact carbohydrates have on blood sugar levels. Protein and fats are excluded from that database since they do not increase blood sugar levels. This is another reason for the emergence of many low-carb diets, such as Dr. Atkins'. 77% of insulin secretion happens independently from glucose levels, though. Insulin production is triggered by incretin. Incretin is a hormone that is produced in the stomach when food is orally consumed. Subsequently, intravenous injections, that bypass the stomach, show no production of incretin. Incretin amounts for 50% to 70% of insulin secrection. Even calorie-free sugars that do not raise blood sugar levels, will lead to a rise in insulin just due to the production of incretin. Therefore, replacing table sugar with calorie-free alternatives or carbohydrates with excessive amounts of protein will not make you lose weight.

Whey protein deserves special consideration in this context, since it strongly stimulates incretin with an increase of 298%, and subsequentally, an insulin production far greater than that of whole-wheat bread. On the other hand, satiety is high after eating whey and feeling full suppresses appetite. Incretin slows down stomach emptying, allowing for your food to sit longer in the stomach. 20% of cow milk consists of whey protein, with casein making up the remaining 80%.[92] Pure fats do not stimulate insulin or glucose levels. This is one of the reasons why popular drinks like *bulletproof coffees* have emerged in recent years. Bulletproof coffee is a cup of black coffee with ghee or butter and MCT (medium-chain triglyceride) oil. Since fat doesn't trigger insulin release, you stay in a ketogenic state.

Last, but not least, high protein and fat consumption lead to fat storage in the body versus usage for conversion into body heat, as it is the case when carbohydrates are mainly consumed. In the China Study, even the least active rural Chinese ate an average of 600 calories *more* and still was slimmer than the average American. Their diet is low in protein and fats, allowing for less fat storage and more active usage of calories.[93]

Lesson 17

Cow milk – yay or nay?

Have you ever wondered why humans are the only species that drink milk after weaning, and in addition to that, from a different species? Cow milk is meant to put hundreds of pounds on calves in a matter of months, made possible through growth hormones in the milk. The dairy industry, however, succeeded in an advertising campaign that praised the health benefits of cow milk, often supported through scientific publications funded by themselves. Nowadays, cows have been genetically so far improved that they continue to lactate throughout the majority of the pregnancy. During pregnancy their sex hormones estrogen and progesterone are significantly higher, though, with higher concentrations of female reproductive hormones making it into the milk. Cow milk consumption can be linked to acne, sexual maturation of prepubertal children, diminished reproductive hormone levels in young men, as well as decreased testosterone secretion. Maybe even more shockingly will be the impact milk consumption may have on women trying to get pregnant: the rate of twin births is five times higher in vegetarians and omnivores consuming cow milk versus milk-abstinent vegan women. IGF, the insulin-like growth factor, is a protein that is released in response to growth hormone and increases ovulation. The IGF concentration in vegan women is 13% lower than in women consuming dairy. The growth hormones in cow milk can stimulate in humans the growth of cancers and certain hormone-sensitive tumors. A meta-analysis (the analyses of a combination of multiple scientific studies) from 2015 concluded that daily high intakes of dairy products, such as milk, low-fat milk, dairy calcium but not supplemental or non-dairy calcium, may increase prostate cancer risk. Researchers dripped milk on human prostate cancer cells in a petri dish to find that the growth of these cancer cells was stimulated. An average increase of more than 30% was reported. Almond milk, on the other hand, was shown to suppress growth of the cancer cells by more than 30%.[94]

A remarkable report from 1992 showed the link between cow milk and type 1 diabetes in children. Type 1 diabetes is an autoimmune disease where the body destroys its own pancreas cells, leading to insufficient or no insulin production. It is believed that undigested proteins that leak into the bloodstream are the cause for some intolerances, allergies and autoimmune diseases. In the study, researchers obtained the blood samples of 142 diabetic children between the age of four and twelve and 79 healthy children. They measured the antibody levels of bovine serum albumin, the cow milk protein believed to be incompletely digested and leaking into the blood stream. Each and every diabetic child had antibody levels higher than 3.55 IgG while all the healthy children had levels below that threshold. There was no overlap between healthy and sick children, leading to the assumption that the diabetic children must have consumed more cow milk and that there might be causation between cow milk and type 1 diabetes. Over the next decades more factors contributing to the development of type 1 diabetes came to light. A study from Chile showed a greater risk for genetically susceptible children that develop the disease when breast-fed for less than three months and weaned too early onto formula based on cow-milk. Under these circumstances, children are 13.1 times (or 1,200%) more likely to develop type 1 diabetes compared to infants breast-fed for at least three months and without these genes. The prevalence of type 1 diabetes is shown to be greater when consumption of cow milk and dairy products is greater. Japan, for instance, has traditionally very few dairy products in their traditional diet while Finland is known to consume the largest amounts of dairy products. Data shows that children in Finland are 36 times more likely to develop type 1 diabetes compared to Japanese children.[95]

With milk alternatives widely available nowadays, it makes it easy to replace cow milk easily in your diet.

Lesson 18

Sugar basics and the glycemic index

Since sugar is believed to be the main culprit in the development of diseases and obesity, this book would not be complete if we didn't look into what makes sugar actually a threat to your health. Let us start with some basics. Glucose is a monosaccharide, or simple sugar, that can be used in every cell in the body. Glucose is sugar circulating in our bloodstream. The excess glucose can be stored as glycogen in the liver and when needed re-converted via a process called gluconeogenesis into glucose. Fructose is another simple sugar naturally found in fruit with a slightly different molecular structure to glucose. While glucose's basic molecular structure is a six-sided ring, fructose's is a five-sided ring. Only the liver can metabolize fructose; muscles and the brain cannot use fructose directly for energy. It does not circulate in the bloodstream, and therefore, blood glucose levels are not notably affected by fructose consumption. Sucrose, also commonly known as "table sugar", is composed of one molecule of glucose linked to one molecule of fructose. Sucrose consists to 50% of fructose and 50% glucose. High fructose corn syrup, for instance, comprises of 55% fructose and 45% glucose. Sucrose naturally occurs in fruits, vegetables and nuts. It is also manufactured from sugar cane and sugar beets. Simple carbohydrates contain a single sugar or two sugars, also called disaccharides. Long chains of hundreds or thousands of sugars linked together are called polysaccharides and are referred to as complex carbohydrates. For the longest time, it was believed that complex carbohydrates let the blood sugar rise gradually due to its digestion taking longer than complex sugar chains. In fact, this is not always the case. White bread, for instance, which is composed of long sugar molecule chains still causes an instant spike in blood glucose levels – just like whole wheat bread! Don't get me wrong, I would still pick whole wheat bread over white bread due to its fiber content. Still, either bread will let the blood sugar rise drastically.

As mentioned earlier, the glycemic index cannot reflect how fructose is affecting insulin levels, only blood sugar levels are measured. Consumption of large amounts of fructose lead in the long run to a fatty liver, which in turn leads to persistently high insulin levels and insulin resistance. High insulin levels lead to persistently high weight. When we look at sucrose now, it becomes evident that both of its components play into the development of insulin resistance: glucose effects insulin rise in the short-term, as reflected in the glycemic index, and then feeds into fructose's long-term impact, once a fatty liver develops.[96]

These are all worst-case scenarios that can happen if no interventions take place. It is never too late to implement healthy habits, even if it is just eating more vegetable/fruits/legumes/whole grains.

Lesson 19

Alternative and artificial sugars and why they aren't better

After science managed to establish in the heads of consumers, that sugar was bad, the food industry started a new quest to find "healthier" alternatives. The industry tapped into natural sources like agave nectar and stevia. Agave nectar occurs naturally in the agave plant and even though it has a low glycemic index, it consists to 80% of fructose. Stevia is extracted from the leaves of Stevia rebaudiana and is 50 to 350 times as sweet as regular sugar. It does not contain fructose and seems to not affect insulin levels.

Below you can find a list of sugars raising insulin levels:

acesulfame potassium (Ace-K™, Sunette™)
Agave
barley syrup
cane juice
cane syrup
corn syrup
fructose
fruit juice concentrate
high fructose corn syrup
honey
malt syrup
maltitol
maple syrup
molasses

monk fruit
rice syrup
saccharine
sorbitol
succanat
sucralose
turbinado
white and brown sugar
xylitol

Sorbitol and xylitol should be enjoyed in small quantities only and are used commercially in mints and chewing gums mainly. Both sweeteners cannot be absorbed by the body, thus, they end up in the colon where they draw in fluid and can cause diarrhea when consumed in large quantities.

Aspartame is another artificial sugar that should be treated with caution. Although it does not raise insulin levels, it seems to have an adverse effect on the gut microbiome and glucose regulation in the liver when taken over extended periods of time. Aspartame and saccharine are associated with a higher risk for depression among older adults. In 1987 the first concern over aspartame's effect on the neurology and behavior of people became public.[97] In 1993 this belief was furthered when a study on subjects with a history of depression had to be halted due to the severe reaction to the artificial sweetener.[98] 2014 brought more clarity on individuals without mental illnesses when a group of adults were split into two groups: one group was given the equivalent of three liters of Diet Coke (the higher dose) for eight days, while the other group received the lower dose, equivalent to one liter of Diet Coke for eight days. Two weeks passed before the groups switched.[99] The FDA recommends not to exceed 50 mg per kilogram body weight per day in aspartame. If you calculate the amounts safe for consumption of aspartame for an average 70 kg or 154 lbs. person, that equals 16 cans (12 oz or 355 ml) per day.[100] The group consuming the higher dose of aspartame consumed about half the acceptable amount as determined by the FDA. Even on half of the acceptable amount, as determined by the FDA, participants were more irritable, exhibited more depression and performed worse on spatial orientation tests. Working memory, however, was not affected.[101] Aspartame is commonly used in sodas and prepared foods. It also goes under the names NutraSweet, Equal and Canderel.

Erythritol or Erythrit is a sugar substitute that has no calories and does not trigger insulin release. It is a sugar alcohol that can naturally occur when things like wine, beer and cheese ferment. It has similar properties to sugar and thus, makes a great substitute for conventional sugar but without harmful side effects like cavities, headaches, fibromyalgia (pain in various muscles and other soft tissue), hypertension or brain disorders, as associated with other artificial sweeteners.

Still, the use of alternatives should be enjoyed with caution. In general, the problem with sweeteners that have no calories is that the brain expects calories but is left with no reward for the sweet taste, potentially leading to cravings. In MRI brain scans, it is visible how glucose fully activates the brain's reward center while artificial sweeteners like sucralose do not have this effect. This could lead to sweet cravings in an attempt to fully activate the reward center, and thus, a habit of eating sweet foods establishes itself. After all, most research shows that no caloric reduction is achieved in test subjects consuming artificial sweeteners.[102]

One fasting day per week can be a great habit to re-set the taste buds and get off the habit of eating sweeter and sweeter treats. You will notice that fasting positively affects the receptors for saltiness just as much, allowing you to use less of both, sugar and salt.

Lesson 20

600 grams (1.3 lbs. or 21.2 oz) of vegetables
400 grams (0.88 lbs. or 14.1 oz) of fruits
100 grams (0.22 lbs. or 3.5 oz) of legumes

Roman challenged us to try and eat 600 grams of vegetables (ideally 300g from above ground raw and 300g from below ground cooked), 400 grams of fruits (100g red peel, 100g green peel, 100g orange/yellow peel and 100g blue/purple peel) and 100 grams of legumes in one day and see how we feel.

My first step in this challenge was the purchase of a food scale. Due to my lack of understanding that eyeballing food sizes led to my overeating, I never got a food scale. The challenge and the importance of strictly following the re-feeding diet forced me to purchase one. It turned out to be the best investment for my long-term success. Understanding portion sizes finally allowed me to stop overeating. Once out of the re-feeding phase, I took up Roman's challenge, at that point without incorporating the 100g of legumes. I couldn't succeed at first! Several things came to play here. Those three food groups are extremely dense in nutrients. My main problem was with ingesting 600g of vegetables per day, though. It takes a very long time to chew them, unlike rice, pasta or bread, you cannot just swallow a spinach leaf or a carrot; you will choke on it. All of a sudden, I spent way more time eating then what I was accustomed to. Midway through my salad, my jaw would start hurting from all the chewing.

Three studies, comprising of six elementary schools, six middle school and six high schools showed that on average only between seven to ten minutes are spent eating lunch in school cafeterias, not taking into account socializing.[103] I started to observe this at work over lunch, as well. My lunch group had finished their cafeteria meal (often a mix of refined carbs, protein and very little vegetable) within ten minutes of us sitting down while it took me three times as long to get through my salad (and most days I wouldn't be able to finish at all). Chewing is the first step of digestion. Saliva contains enzymes that help break down carbohydrates and make them more easily absorbed in the gut. However, it takes the brain approximately 20 minutes to signal satiation from a meal. If you scarf down your food in seven to ten minutes, you will still feel hungry. It was visible to me in my lunch group: my colleagues left the table hungry! By picking a meal that takes you more than 20 minutes to eat, you will slow down eating and reach fullness after your meal.

At first, I still combined the suggested amounts of vegetables and fruits with whole grain bread/pasta/rice and meat/fish/sea food. After all, didn't we learn that carbs are an important part of each meal? Remember, I didn't incorporate 100g of legumes at that point. I realized very soon that I could leave out the carbs and still be full. The high-fiber content of these foods provides volume and fullness over a long period of time without ingesting many calories. The only problem I noticed was that due to my gut bacteria not being used to the high volumes of vegetables, in particular the fiber, I constantly felt bloated. A better approach for me was to include the legumes and complex carbs and gradually increase vegetable amounts. It also helped me to take probiotic capsules. They helped to build my good gut bacteria and digest the fiber. Learning to incorporate legumes in my daily diet added a great benefit to feel full over a long period of time.

A weight loss study impressively demonstrated how legumes help with slimming down and getting healthier contrary to just cutting calories. A group of overweight subjects were divided into two groups: the first group had to incorporate five cups of legumes per week without changing their diet in any other way, while the second group was asked to cut out 500 calories per day. Not only did the first group lose weight, their blood sugar levels, insulin function and cholesterol improved.[104]

Another intervention study on overweight subjects confirms the finding that eating as much as you want of mainly plant-based whole foods, and low-fat leads to weight loss. In this particular study, the study subjects lost an average of 17 pounds in three weeks. Let me repeat this: by eating as much as they wanted, but of the right foods, overweight people *lost* weight.[105] These results are not unique. They were recreated in similar studies with similar success rates. The only times, this approach will not work is when too many refined grains, like pasta, rice and pastries, remain in the diet. Replacing meat with dairy will also not yield the same weight-loss result.[106]

Lesson 21

Fiber – the skeleton of plants

Studies have shown that high fiber intake not only seems to reduce the risk of various cancers and diseases but also can prevent strokes, dementia and Alzheimer's disease. Most Americans, unfortunately, only eat an average of 15 g of fiber a day, instead of the recommended 25 g for women and 38 g for men.

Your fiber intake can prevent cardiovascular diseases, like strokes. Strokes are caused by ruptured plaques in the arteries that sever blood flow to parts of the brain; similar to heart attacks that cut off blood flow to the heart. Alzheimer's disease is a form of dementia and unlike strokes and heart attacks, plague the sufferer and people close to them progressively over an extended period of time. The two identified reasons are amyloid plaques, a protein deposit, that clogs the brain tissue itself, and the tangle of neurofibrillary; both lead to the death of brain cells and subsequentially the shrinkage of the affected brain region. Symptoms depend on the stage the affected person is in but include memory loss, cognitive problems, impaired reasoning or judgment and repeating questions, just to list a few.

The exact workings of fiber on the brain are not clear but it could be the combination of fiber's positive effects on controlling cholesterol and blood sugar levels which help reduce the risk of artery clogs. Diets rich in fiber seem to promote lower blood pressure which in turn lowers the risk of brain bleeds. More importantly, fiber binds toxins in the body, such as lead and mercury. Unwanted waste products like excess cholesterol and estrogen are all deposited in the intestines and would normally be discarded with stool but when insufficient amounts of fiber are consumed, the unwanted waste products can be re-absorbed. The body's effort to detoxify is undermined.[107]

Intermittent fasting, every-other-day fasting, fasting one day a week or fasting cures all have an anti-aging effect by allowing the body to get into autophagy and in that way, start the self-eating/cleaning process. Scientists were already able to show in rats that every-other-day fasting increased their lifespan; their nerve cells were better protected and kept functioning longer. Further, mice fed a high-fiber diet had reduced inflammation in the immune cells of their brain, the so-called microglia.[108] Cognitive decline with age is believed to be caused by inflammation in microglia. The challenge lies once again in finding willing human subjects to stick with the restrictive eating windows over an extended period of time to make these findings applicable to humans.

The intake of probiotic capsules and prebiotics or, where possible, foods and beverages containing natural pro- and prebiotics help digest fiber. Roman stressed the importance of good bacteria in the gut for not only better digestion but also immunity, physical and mental health. My major lessons learned surrounding digestion, the gut brain and gut bacteria will follow later in the book.

Lesson 22

Ingredient lists and additives – why shorter is better

The major lesson here is that the shorter the list of added ingredients, the better the product probably is for your health. The most eye-opening example Roman gave was cheese. Up to that moment, I had never looked at the ingredients of cheese, and had I done so before, I wouldn't have understood much. The least ingredients needed to make cheese are: milk, salt and rennet. Rennet is a set of enzymes that can be found in the stomach lining of young ruminants (animals that chew the cud; specifically herbivorous, even-toed, hoofed mammals). Cheese that is not made completely naturally includes cornstarch and E numbers (additives used to enhance flavor, texture, color and preservability), like calcium chloride. Cheese made with raw milk has the added benefit of naturally occurring good bacteria. Pasteurized milk is heated to kill harmful organisms that can cause disease in humans and most dairy products you will find in supermarkets are produced with pasteurized milk for reasons of food safety.

The one organization that self-declared as their mission to protect *"the public health by ensuring the safety, efficacy, and security of human and veterinary drugs, biological products, and medical devices; and by ensuring the safety of our nation's food supply, cosmetics, and products that emit radiation"*, the US Food and Drug Administration (FDA) has questionable standards for ensuring public health.[109] One of their labels, the "generally recognized as safe" (GRAS) status is, in fact, given to additives by their manufacturers. Yes, you read correctly. This is a status the FDA deems not to require government or scientific body approval; the company manufacturing the product self-determinates its safety for the public. To make things even worse, the FDA does not have to be notified about added ingredients to the food supply by the manufacturer. Thousands of decisions on food-additive safety have never been reported to the FDA or the public. However, some new additives are voluntarily reported to the FDA by manufacturers. Unfortunately, none of the entities reporting these additives are independent from the manufacturer; in fact, between 1997 and 2012 the voluntarily submitted GRAS safety determinations were coming from the following sources:

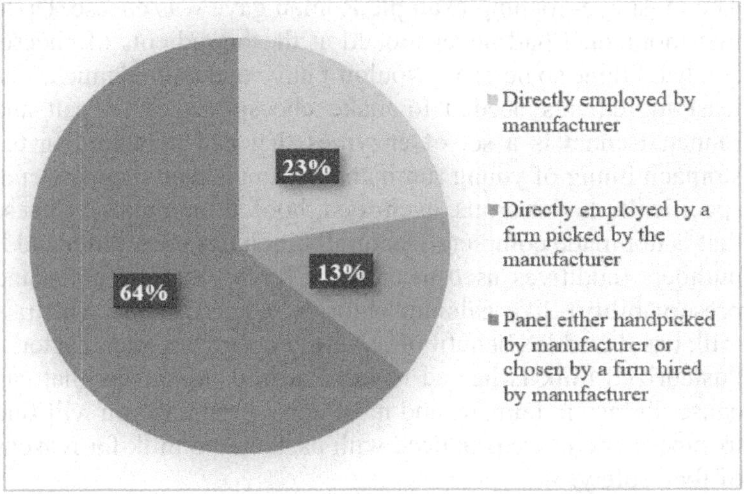

It won't come to anyone's surprise that three of Washington's largest lobbying companies work for the food industry, neither that many members of scientific boards and panels – boards and panels that are supposed to give nutritional advice to the public – receive some sort of monetary compensation from meat, dairy, egg and agriculture associations.

Common preservatives in cured meat, like bacon, sausage, ham, salami and hot dogs, are nitrite and nitrate. Nitrite is an additive that gives cured meats its pink color. In addition, it inhibits the growth of harmful bacteria. Nitrate can be found concentrated in green, leafy vegetables and beets, and is generally considered good for human health. Your body can convert the nitrate into nitric oxide which allows for better oxygen transportation and blood flow to the heart. In contrast, if you lack nitric oxide or the nitric-oxide-producing enzyme is inhibited, your arteries can stiffen, leading to dysfunctions that cause blood pressure to rise and the risk of heart attacks to increase. At the same time, the nitrate that naturally occurs in vegetables can be fermented into nitrite. Nitrite can turn into the carcinogens nitrosamines and nitrosamides when exposed to amines and amides, as found plentifully in animal protein. This process can either happen in the meat itself or when digested in your stomach. However, when a plant is the source of the nitrate, the accompanying vitamin C and antioxidants of the whole food block the carcinogenic compound from forming in the body.

Nitrosamines and nitrosamides are by-products of cigarette smoke. Cigarette smoke is so potent, it can remain in a room even when the room is ventilated by sticking to walls and fabrics. A study from 2007 linked cured meat consumption to higher risks of chronic obstructive pulmonary disease (COPD). Uncured meats are at times advertised as nitrite or nitrate free with a footnote "except those naturally occurring in celery juice". Knowing that the nitrate from fermented celery juice can turn into nitrite, and this in turn reacts with animal protein to form toxic nitrosamines and nitrosamides, is a crooked method to deceive consumers. A higher risk of kidney cancer is associated with exposure to nitrosamines and nitrosamides, while vegetables rich in nitrate work to reduce such cancer risk.

Another food additive that should be steered clear of is phosphate. There is no need to restrict the intake of phosphorus that naturally occurs as a mineral in plants, in the form of phytate, since the mineral is incompletely absorbed by the body. In animals, however, phosphorus appears in the form of a compound called phosphate. Contrary to the plant's phytate, phosphate is much more eagerly absorbed into the bloodstream and can have adverse effects on health when alleviated levels are prevalent. High serum phosphate concentrations can contribute to kidney failure, heart failure, heart attacks and premature death, in addition to blood vessel damage, accelerated aging and bone loss. The average American adult ingests almost double of the recommended dietary allowance for phosphorus, mainly due to the phosphate added to processed foods. Phosphate food additives are used to preserve moisture and color, as well as, enhance and stabilize frozen foods. They are added to enhance the color of meat and drinks like Coca-Cola. In the food industry it is common to inject chicken with phosphate salts to improve the color, add water weight (salt binds water) and reduce loss of liquid from ageing meat. A publication in 2009 revealed, though, that eight of the 25 uncooked meat and poultry products that used additives did not report those on the label. In the US, there is no requirement to include phosphorus or potassium content on nutrition labels.[110] The practice of injecting raw meat and poultry with phosphate salts has been long banned in the European Union with the understanding that consumer protection requires the disclosure of additives, such as phosphate salts, that can endanger the health of patients with renal (kidney) disease and those on dialysis.[111] In the US, on the other hand, eleven different types of phosphate salts are permitted. High phosphate levels are the reason for increased cardiovascular risk and mortality which lead to impaired arterial function within hours of consumption. Even more worrisome becomes added phosphate in meat. This additive may increase the growth of Campylobacter, a bacteria strain found in poultry that is linked to food poisoning in humans.[112]

While all the allowed additives in the food industry are assumed to be safe for consumers, there are instances where allowed amounts of an additive are only limited to that particular product; meaning, that you could still overconsume on an additive because the regulated numbers on the label refer to one particular product only, not the entirety of your diet. If your diet mainly consists of processed foods, there is a good chance you are overconsuming – and absorbing – phosphate. Therefore, as much as possible, stay away from processed foods!

Lesson 23

Ingredient lists and sodium amounts

Sodium intake is closely linked to high blood pressure. Salt binds water which leads to water retentions, when large amounts are consumed. In order to get rid of the excess water, your body raises its blood pressure. Studies have shown that people with high-blood pressure that are put on sodium-low diets, can see their blood pressure drop. The daily recommendation for sodium intake by the American Heart Association is less than 1,500 mg per day, or ¾ of a teaspoon. However, the average American adult ingests between 2,900 and 4,300 mg daily – more than double! Chronic high salt intake leads to a gradual surge in a person's blood pressure over the span of their lifetime.

While doctors believed that a rise in blood pressure is normal with age, a study in the Amazonian tribe of the Yanomamo presented a different picture. The Yanomamo have the lowest ever recorded sodium intake and with that not a single case of high blood pressure recorded. They mainly eat a plant-based diet and exercise a lot. Before the invention of pills, malignant hypertension, one of the most severe forms of high blood pressure, was a death sentence with a life expectancy of approximately six months. Nowadays, instead of telling people to change their diet, they are prescribed pills. Further studies into the effect of high sodium consumption, showed that blood flow becomes impaired, thus, affecting arterial function. Vitamin C injections into the skin showed to reverse much of the damage, leading to the conclusion that oxidative stress is the reason for the suppression of blood vessel function. Later on, it was found that superoxide dismutase, a key antioxidant enzyme in the body that can detoxify millions of free radicals per second, is suppressed with sodium intake. Harmful levels of oxidative stress can build up this way.[113] This could be the explanation for why you should drink a large glass of lukewarm lemon water first thing in the morning – get the vitamin C in before any sodium is consumed!

With salt's property of retaining water, it quickly attracted the interest of the food industry: after all, they could easily add weight to their products without actually providing more nutrients. And so, manufacturers started to add salt to meat, increasing the products weight by up to 20%. As mentioned previously, chicken carcasses are injected with salt water, artificially increasing their weight while being allowed to still label the product as 100% natural. The greatest sodium contributor to diet for ages 20 to 50 is chicken – not potato chips, canned soups or pretzels.[114]

Sodium derivatives are contained in flavor enhancers, thickeners, preservatives or texture enhancers. On ingredient lists they will be labelled as disodium guanylate, disodium inosinate, disodium ethylenediaminetetraacetic acid (EDTA) sodium caseinate, sodium benzoate, sodium bicarbonate and sodium nitrite, just to list a few. If you can't avoid buying processed foods, try to limit the sodium intake by buying foods with fewer mg of sodium than there are grams in the serving size. For example, the serving size of regular ketchup is 17 g. Ideally, sodium should be less than 17 mg. Unfortunately, though, 17 g of Ketchup contain 180 mg of sodium.

Natural foods lowering blood pressure that have been scientifically proven to work are flaxseeds and hibiscus tea. Eating flaxseeds unknowingly over six months every day, significantly lowered the blood pressure of participants almost two to three times better than some of the most powerful antihypertensive drugs on the market. Two strong cups of hibiscus tea every morning, not exceeding five tea bags, had similarly beneficial effects in a group taking starting doses of the drug Captopril twice a day.[115]

One remarkable side effect of the 10-day fast, was the reduced salt intake I experienced afterwards. Salt-taste receptors become more sensitive, allowing for smaller amounts to be added to food while not feeling like you are compromising on flavor. The weekly fasts of 36-hours aid in keeping sodium intake low. Taste buds acclimate to levels of exposure, requiring higher amounts over time, therefore a re-set day might be exactly what your body needs.

Lesson 24

A basic lesson in digestion and its link to food allergies, gluten, lactose and fructose intolerance

We cannot solely focus on diet and nutrition, without looking into what happens with the different foods once they enter our system. For that reason, digestion, the link to our health, both physical and mental, has to be understood first.

Let's start by looking at how food is digested. After chewing and swallowing that first bite of your meal, it will land in the stomach for its next processing stage. Stomach acid is released to kill any harmful substances and break down the foods further. Muscles of the gastric wall contract and throw the content off its walls. Simple carbohydrates are passed quickly to the small intestine while fats and proteins remain longer in the stomach to be broken down further. The next stop is the small intestine. With a length of 16.4 to 19.7 feet (5 to 6 meters), the small intestine is covered with thousands of intestinal villi and microvilli (the villi on top of the villi) which extract nutrients from food. If all the villi were ironed out to a smooth surface, the small intestine would be roughly 4.5 miles (7 km) long![116] The reason is that our body needs to break down everything you eat to the smallest possible size until it can be absorbed into your cells – you literally become what you eat. Digestive enzymes and fat solvents are produced by the liver and pancreas to extract fat, protein (the amino acids in particular) and sugar; fiber, which is indigestible by the small intestine, is passed to the large intestine. The large intestine is approximately 3.3 to 5 feet long (1 to 1.5 meters) and wraps around the small intestine. Most of the gut bacteria is found in the walls of the large intestine where it breaks down the last nutritious substances; a process that can take as long as 16 hours. Here water and salt are extracted from the chyme and mucus is mixed into what becomes the feces. The rectum stores the feces when relieving oneself is not immediately possible.

One part of the large intestine is the appendix, located below the junction between small and large intestine and completely isolated from the action of digesting food. For many years it was believed that the appendix, as well as tonsils, are a useless, at times even bothersome, organ. The appendix, when inflamed, causes a lot of pain and has to be urgently surgically removed. Untreated appendicitis will cause the appendix to burst, leading to more inflammation and subsequently to death.

Just like the tonsils in your mouth, the appendix is part of the tonsillar immune tissue. The appendix is almost entirely made of immune tissue and its main purpose is to eliminate bad bacteria so that only good germs remain.

Many theories surrounding the cause of food allergies and intolerances – from gluten, lactose and fructose – focus on the role digestion plays. In food allergies, one assumption is that the amino acids of a protein, for instance the peanut, are not broken down enough in the small intestine. This tiny particle that remains undigested can end up in the lymphatic system, embedded in fat droplets. Normally only fats and fat-soluble vitamins from the gut are making it into the lymphatic system for circulation in the veins. The ever so vigilant immune cells know the permitted substances in the lymphatic system, detect the foreign object and start eliminating it by attacking the intruder. If this happens frequently enough, the immune system's response becomes better and faster and over time more aggressive. At some point, putting a peanut in your mouth, will cause such a severe allergic reaction, that your lips, tongue and throat will swell up almost instantly. The explanation provided applies to foods rich in fat and protein in general, like milk, eggs and peanuts.

With gluten it is important to differentiate between gluten intolerance, a genetical predisposition affecting one in a hundred people, and gluten sensitivity, meaning gluten causes some digestive discomfort and unpleasant immune reaction but can be consumed in moderate amounts. The actual gluten intolerance, called celiac disease, can damage the villi of the small intestine, cause serious infections and in some cases also damage the nervous system. 99% of wheat grown worldwide is a dwarf or semi-dwarf variant that was created in in the 50s to accomplish higher-yield wheat. Further tweaks led to today's variants that yield great outputs but unfortunately lack in micronutrient content. One explanation for why gluten is not always well digested by people lies in the grains, trying to protect its seeds from being consumed by animals and humans; after all, their reproduction relies on the seed making it back into the ground. Therefore, plants make their seeds slightly poisonous. In grasshoppers, for instance, an important digestive enzyme is inhibited when wheat is consumed. Even though most humans are not affected by these seeds, it can happen that due to a porous gut, the undigested wheat finds its way into the cells of the gut where it can loosen the connection between individual cells. Once again, a foreign body enters areas it has no business in, triggering a reaction by the immune system. Another explanation for the prevalence of celiac disease could be Western diets predominantly relying on wheat as its main source. After all, no generation before ours had to digest the amounts we expect our gut to process.

Lactose intolerance, by contrast, is not a real intolerance but rather a deficiency of a required digestive enzyme that breaks down the chemical bond between the two sugar molecules of lactose. Unlike gluten, undigested lactose does not travel through the gut wall but passes on to the large intestine where the gas-producing bacteria are feasting on it. Most humans are born with the enzyme to break down lactose. As people get older, the gene to digest lactose, however, begins to switch off in 75% of people. The level of lactose-splitting enzymes is gradually reduced but commonly enough enzymes are available to digest smaller amounts. Humans were never meant to consume dairy products once they are not breastfed anymore – contrary to the belief of the dairy industry.

In people with hereditary intolerance to fructose, fewer enzymes to process sugar exist. In people that develop a fructose intolerance later in life, the problem lies in the absorption of fructose. It seems like fewer transporters are available leading to the undigested sugar passing to the large intestine where it feeds the gut bacteria causing bloating. The result is an unbalanced gut flora. We mentioned fructose before and how the consumed amounts have significantly increased in recent years. Fructose intolerance nowadays seems to stem from eating too large amounts of this sugar. Researchers discovered that untreated fructose malabsorption over a long period of time can lead to depression. The reason is how tryptophan and fructose interact during digestion. The amino acid tryptophan is a neurotransmitter responsible for producing serotonin, the "happiness hormone". Serotonin has a calming effect, stimulates cognitive performance, aids sleep and makes one feel full after a meal. During digestion tryptophan latches on to fructose. When absorption of fructose is dysfunctional, the sugar, as well as the attached tryptophan are lost. Symptoms of serotonin deficiency can be bad mood, anxiety and aggression.

Even in people who are not fructose intolerant, eating large amounts of this sugar can lead to the suppression of leptin, the hormone making you feel full.[117]

Lesson 25

The Gut Brain and why what we eat can make us depressed – prisoners

In 1997, a correctional facility in California, USA, decided to give its prisoners the choice between two paths. One was the so-called "New Start" program. It constituted of a vegan diet in combination with bible studies, occupational training and anger management. Alternatively, inmates could continue to receive the standard high carbohydrates "prison food" diet. At that time, the recidivism rate was a whopping 95%. To the surprise of many, 85% of the 500 inmates agreed to live in the wing of the prison that offered a vegan menu and the rehabilitation program. What was presented to them was unbelievable: while the wing that housed the 15% of inmates that did not want to participate experienced racial tension, fights and gang terrain, prisoners of New Start were fully racially integrated, calmer, smiled more, made better decisions, eagerly attended the offered program and cooperated more. The biggest success, though, was the drop in the recidivism rate from 95% to 2%. Even though the facility was shut down after seven years due to a miscellaneous dispute, the impact this experiment left, did not vanish.[118]

The gut brain, also referred to as the second brain, is a network of nerves, rivaling in complexity and size the brain's system. While the brain operates on a conscious level through sensory organs like the skin, eyes, ears and nose, the gut brain gives a picture of the inside, using the huge surface area of the comprised digestive system, working subconsciously on the mind. Even though we have no conscious control over processes of the gut, it is connected to particular parts of the brain and thus, influences our thinking, mood and behavior. Signals from the gut, for instance, can reach the following areas of the brain and in simplified terms, their respective responsibility:

Insula

- Self-awareness

Limbic system

- Emotions

Prefrontal cortex

- Morality

Amygdala

- Fear

Hippocampus

- Memory

Anterior cingulate cortex

- Motivation

The most direct and fastest route between brain and gut is the *nervus vagus*, or vagus nerve. The gut is in the midst of the action inside you and has all the information on your organs, hormones, activity of immune cells, your last meal. Information is processed in the gut brain and if deemed important, transmitted to the brain that sits safe and insolated in the skull, embedded in a thick membrane. The brain, on the other hand, does not allow for all information to pass; it assesses if the data is important enough to be registered. For example, when you walk in a park on a warm summer day, there will be an overload of outside stimuli, from the temperature your skin perceives, to the various sounds of birds, humans, cars, planes, as well as smells and visual cues. Not all of them will make it to your conscious brain though. The brain filters what is important to process the environment in order for you to react appropriately. The same applies to your gut brain. Information is screened and assessed before transmission. An inconspicuous apple you just ate will not make it from the gut to the brain. Satiation from food will make it to the brain, as well as discomfort after a meal. The vagus nerve detects inflammation in the body which it communicates to the brain. As a response, your body gears up the immune system, inhibiting inflammation. The vagus nerve seems to work in the opposite direction of chronic inflammation. By stimulation, through deep breathing or connecting with people, it can be strengthened just like a muscle.

A revealing experiment in mice showed how powerful the gut is when it comes to mental health. Mice were put in the following situation: a container was filled with water to the extent where the mice could not reach the bottom anymore. The scientists wanted to see how long the mice would continue to swim, in hope of hitting land, before they give up. A mouse with depressive tendencies does not last long; its motivational drive seems to be inhibited. The same depressed mice react stronger to stress. One way to test the effectiveness of antidepressant medicine, is to see if these depressed rodents will swim longer when given the drugs. In a next step, the mice were divided in two groups: one group was given *Lactobacillus rhamnosus*, a bacteria strain known for its beneficial effect on the gut, while the other group remained on the same diet. The result was that not only did the group with the better gut flora swim longer, motivated to survive, they also showed fewer stress hormones in their blood and displayed better cognitive and learning abilities compared to their peers. A severed *nervus vagus*, however, leveled the field. Once the information cannot make it from the gut to the brain, the good bacteria strain had no effect.

Two years after the experiment on mice, researchers altered the gut flora of humans with the remarkable result of an altered brain, in particular the areas responsible for processing emotions and pain. Chinese researchers were also able to show that *Lactobacillus reuteri* inhibits pain sensors in the gut. Pain therapy can entail replenishing your gut flora with good gut bacteria.

Earlier stress was discussed in relation to how cortisol affects blood sugar levels and insulin. Let's look now at how stress affects the gut. In a stressful situation, the brain needs energy to solve the problem so it tells the gut to hold its operations. The gut obliges, blood supply is reduced, less mucus is produced and digestion halted. As a consequence, nutrients are not extracted as efficiently, less energy is absorbed from food and digestion takes longer. Once again, over a short period of time, the body will be able to deal with the stress but the problems arise when the gut is put on a permanent hold. People who are constantly stressed will attest to bad digestion, diarrhea and constipation. With less mucus available and a lower blood supply, the gut walls are left weakened, and the gut bacteria and immune cells more exposed. Mealtime should be early on established as a stress-free down time. Distractions like television or phones should be avoided, as well as scolding or other anxiety-inducing situations.

To study the effects of gut microbiomes, scientists have bred germ-free mice. What sounds at first impossible, is made reality by growing the rodents in sterile isolators where they are kept in antiseptic cages, fed steam-sterilized food and have no connection to the outside world. Their behavior is odd and unlike what can be observed with free-living mice. They exhibit hyperactivity, lack caution, overeat and digest food longer. In addition, their appendixes are enlarged, their digestive tract is shriveled and have only few villi, plus fewer immune cells are available. When fed with the bacteria of mice suffering from type 2 diabetes, something interesting happened: the previously germ-free mice develop problems metabolizing sugar. When administered with the bacteria of obese humans, the mice became more likely to gain weight. These fascinating findings shed light on how important bacteria and its composition are for health.

The first development of our gut flora happens with birth. By going through the birth channel, the child is exposed to the vaginal bacteria of its mother, followed by the bacteria that reside on the skin. All these factors will contribute to the bacteria residing in the gut. Research has shown that babies born via caesarian section are more prone to develop allergies, asthma and food intolerances later in life. However, when these babies are administered *Lactobacillus*, the risk of developing allergies is reduced. At the same time, this treatment makes no difference in babies born naturally.

As an adult, nutrition, the use of antibiotics, level of cleanliness and exposure to certain bacteria will influence the composition of your gut bacteria.[119]

Lesson 26

Gut bacteria and how it influences our immunity

The big lesson here is that 80% of your immunity lies in your gut.

Our gut microbiome and body are in a symbiotic relationship. The gut microbiome is an ecosystem of its own consisting of approximately 100 trillion bacteria (this is way more than we have of human cells!) which are home to more than 1,000 different species of bacteria, in addition to smaller populations of viruses, yeasts, fungi and other single-celled organisms. The gut microbiome can weigh up to 2 kg (4.5 lbs). They are responsible for digesting food, producing vitamins, supplying the gut with energy, breaking down toxins and determining our immunity. One might wonder now how these bacteria manage to survive without being attacked by their host. First of all, the bacteria are in a closed-off area on one side of the intestinal lining, the mucus membrane, away from the rest of the digestive tract. It seems like the bacteria manage to make the immune cells believe that they are no threat to the body and will do no harm.

When immature immune cells are produced, they acquaint themselves with the bacteria without posing any danger to the body. That way the immune cells are trained on all the bacteria residing in the gut. As a result, they can react better and quicker when confronted with intruders elsewhere in the body; the immune cells will recognize the bacteria from the previous training and know what to do. Crucial for an immune cell is its ability to distinguish self-produced cells from foreign cells. However, it gets tricky when bacteria are encountered where the surface resembles a human cell. This is the case with scarlet fever and the reason why an immediate antibiotic therapy has to be started before the immune system starts attacking its own tissue.

Type 1 diabetes that develops due to environmental factors can have its cause rooted in the gut bacteria present. In patients with type 1 diabetes, insulin producing cells of the pancreas are destroyed by immune cells, resulting in too little or no insulin production. Clinical studies have shown a decreased diversity of gut bacteria before onset of the disease which remains after type 1 diabetes has been diagnosed.

The composition of the gut microbiome can influence weight. There are bacteria that can extract more energy from meals by breaking down carbohydrates more efficiently. In doing so, more calories are absorbed. Even when two people eat the exact same quantities, the one with more of the energy extracting bacteria will put on weight. One reason for it are the fatty acids that bacteria produce. There are fatty acids that can be metabolized in the gut and liver; those are produced by vegetable-loving bacteria. Other fatty acids feed the rest of the body. You will have heard before that calories are not always calories; that stems from the understanding that the impact of one calorie is different depending on where it comes from. You can eat a banana with x calories and will probably not put on weight compared to eating the same amount of calories in chocolate. The bacteria that break down that banana are able to extract components valuable to certain crucial functions in the body. Researchers found less diversity in the gut flora of obese patients, as well as higher quantities of carbohydrate metabolizing bacteria. This alone is not the reason for weight gain though. The second marker for extreme weight gain scientists found was inflammation. Metabolic problems will show in the blood by slightly increased inflammatory markers. Affected are mostly obese and diabetic patients, as well as people with high levels of triglycerides. Immediate treatment is in these cases not necessary; however, low levels of inflammation, called subclinical infection, do not go unnoticed by your bacteria. Bacteria have a signaling substance on their surface, notifying the body when to get infected. As long as bacteria remain in their mucus-membrane, no inflammatory reaction is triggered; the body will not rid itself from harmful substances. The story looks different though, when bacteria find its way into the bloodstream, through a bad diet, for instance. The signaling substances excreted by bacteria can latch onto organs, like the liver or fatty tissue, and disrupt metabolism from there by promoting the deposition of more fat. Thyroid glands are equally affected by such bacterial infections. The production of sufficient thyroid hormones is blocked leading to a slowed down metabolism which shows itself through inhibited fat burning. Other factors such as hormonal imbalances, vitamin D insufficiency, elevated amounts of estrogen or diets rich in gluten can similarly cause subclinical infections.

In 2013 a new theory was introduced: bacteria cause cravings. What seems at first unconnected makes more sense if you think of bacteria living in the host in symbiosis and the composition of the bacteria depending on what the host eats. If you eat meat regularly, your gut will have the meat-eating bacteria ready for digestion. The other way around the same logic applies, if you, for instance, never eat beans, you will not have the bacteria available to digest beans. In many people, eating beans irregularly will lead to bloating. Bacteria, like any other living organism, want to survive. One means of survival researchers believe they use, is the production of neurotransmitters. The reason lies in how information from the gut brain reaches the brain. Only pure sugar, minerals and neurotransmitters can pass through the blood vessels to the brain. By producing neurotransmitters like tyrosine and tryptophan that in turn build the hormones dopamine and serotonin, our gut bacteria find a way to influence our brain. Dopamine stimulates the reward center in the brain. Serotonin is the hormone that makes us feel happy and positively influences cognitive functions. Studies have shown that a meal rich in nutrients our bacteria like, increases the transmitters signaling satiation. Since most of the bacteria are located in the large intestine, they prefer indigestible foods, like fiber in legumes and vegetables.

Anyone who loves sugary treats, will attest to cravings whenever they go too long without something sweet. I know from experience that these cravings subside. I went numerous times in my life without added sugar for several weeks, just eating naturally occurring sugar from fruits. Could my bacteria that digest sugar be the reason? Could they be starved?

Another interesting observation was made in the 1970s when studies on African Maasai warriors shed more light on the connection between cholesterol and gut bacteria. The tribesmen of Maasai spend about 13 hours a day walking and fast for a month of the year. American scientists were surprised to see that even though the Maasai warriors ate a diet rich in meat and curdled milk, their cholesterol levels were low. Little was understood at that time about curdled, or fermented, milk and how certain bacteria are required to curdle the milk. At that time, the researchers could not make out or recreate the effects they witnessed. Many experiments later with various bacteria cultures, varying quantities and durations of administration, as well as means of administrations on animals first, led to vital discoveries in humans later. In particular, an experiment in 2011 on 114 Canadians provided insight into the influence bacteria have on cholesterol. Test subjects were given twice a day for six weeks a yoghurt with Lactobacillus reuteri which is known to be especially resistant to stomach acid. The bad cholesterol, LDL, sunk by 8.9 %. Taking cholesterol-lowering drugs would have achieved double the reduction in LDL but with side effects. Other combinations of bacteria strains showed even better improvements in cholesterol levels. The major contributing factor seems to lie in bacteria with the ability to convert bile salts. Bile acid, which is stored in the gallbladder, is produced from cholesterol and used for digestion of fatty acids. After it helps with the digestion of fat, it can be almost entirely resorbed in the small intestine. An enzyme built by certain gut bacteria called bile salt hydrolase (BSH), however, can alter bile acid to inhibit the resorption resulting in the excretion with stool. In turn, the liver has to produce more bile acid by using cholesterol available in the blood stream. This shows that cholesterol is important for certain functions in the body and complete avoidance of it is nothing to strive for. Instead, the aim should be consumption of good cholesterol, or HDL, which occurs in fatty fish, nuts, olive oil, whole grains, beans, legumes, chia and flax seeds, just to name a few.

Here a list of bacteria with bile salt hydrolase (BSH) activity:

Bifidobacterium adolescentis	*L. fermentum*
B. animalis	*L. gasseri*
B. breve	*L. helveticus*
B. infantis	*L. paracasei subsp. paracasei*
B. longum	*L. rhamnosus*
Bifidobacterium sp.	*L. plantarum*
Lactobacillus acidophilus	*L. casei*

Researchers observed in healthy and lean people a bigger gut bacteria diversity in comparison to obese people.

When possible, raw milk products, like raw milk butter, yoghurt or cheese, and products with active bacteria cultures, like kombucha or fermented sauerkraut, should be consumed. Of course, due consideration needs to be given when pregnant or breast feeding.[120]

Fasting allows the gut bacteria to reestablish a healthy equilibrium. Bad bacteria in an equilibrium will make you stronger, while the good bacteria will protect you. Fasting gives you the chance to re-populate your gut by eating vegetables, fruits and fibers once solid foods are re-introduced into the diet.

Lesson 27

Probiotics and prebiotics – boost your health

Probiotics are bacteria that are beneficial to your health and can be found in certain foods and beverages while prebiotics are carbohydrates, most often indigestible fiber, that feed good gut bacteria.

Through the process of fermentation, humanity discovered a long time ago a way to preserve foods and beverages. In Germany and Austria, traditionally sauerkraut, pickled gherkin and sourdough bread can be found, in the Balkan region Kaymak (a creamy dairy product), in Eastern Europe Kefir (a fermented yoghurt), Turkey has its yoghurt drink Ayran, Asia has soy sauce, miso paste, kimchi (fermented cabbage), pickled radishes, natto (fermented soybeans), and Switzerland and Italy have their cheeses, just to name a few. The problem we face in the industrialized food industry is that many of the naturally, healthy occurring bacteria strains are killed by pasteurization. It is difficult to guarantee no exposure to dangerous pathogens, thus, one of the safest methods available is treatment with heat. The use of vinegar is another way to create the otherwise naturally occurring sour taste from fermentation in pickles for instance. The consumer is left, once again, with an empty shell of a product, stripped of all its once healthy features.

In the early 1900s the mountain peasants of Bulgaria intrigued one scientist, Ilya Metchnikoff. With fascination he observed the longevity of these people who would live to be 100 years old. He soon discovered that the milk they were carrying for long distances home, started to turn sour in their leather bags. The bacteria strain discovered is called Lactobacillus bulgaricus and was found to be a contributing factor to good health in the peasants.

Good gut bacteria have the following benefits:

Help the villi

- to grow bigger and more robust so that more beneficial nutrients can be absorbed and unhealthy substances dissapated

Starve bad bacteria

- by sntaching away their food

Treat diahrrea

- without any of the potential side effects you might see from drugs;
- it can increase the intervals between diahrrea attacks and flare-ups of inflammation

Train immune system

- to prevent colds, especially in people who are prone to get sick often

Off-set of allergies can be potentially prevented

- especially in childern with potential of developing allergies, e.g. in children born by Cesarean section or not breastfed

If you decide to take probiotics, it is recommended to take them for at least four weeks to see any results. Since the strains you can buy in the pharmacy are isolated, they tend to vanish once you stop taking them. After all, the gut is already densely populated with bacteria and finding a place for someone new can be challenging.[121]

Prebiotics are what feed the good gut bacteria and allow them to grow. Bad bacteria cannot digest prebiotics and thus, do not produce the chemicals that make you crave unhealthy foods. They occur naturally in the following foods, with chicory root providing the highest content of the fiber inulin:

Artichoke	Asparagus	Endive
Green bananas	Jerusalem artichoke	Garlic
Onion	Parsnips	Black salsify
Wholegrain wheat	Rye	Whole oats
Leek	Chicory root	Dandelion greens
Barley	Apples	Konjac root
Cocoa beans	Flaxseeds	Seaweed
Soy beans	Legumes (peas and beans)	Yacon root

Another favorite of the good gut bacteria are resistant starches. Resistant starches cannot be broken down in the small intestine, so, they pass on undigested to the large intestine where they become food for the good gut bacteria. When, for instance potatoes or rice are boiled and then left to cool, the starches crystalize and resistant starch forms. Cold sushi rice is one such healthy example that in addition to containing resistant starches, also is enriched with rice vinegar which promotes fermentation.

Inulin is a dietary fiber and sugar that can be found in many root vegetables. It can be used as a fat or sugar substitute. Mixed with water, inulin becomes gel-like. Roman recommends to replace up to 10% of sugar in a recipe with inulin. Inulin has barely any sweetness, has only one third of the calories of sugar, adds bulk and thus, makes you feel full quicker. Since it is pure fiber not too much should be used, otherwise the texture of the baked goods might become too tough. I can confirm that my chocolate brownies with inulin and erythrite, which is a sugar substitute that is almost calorie free and does not trigger the blood sugar, taste great and keep their texture.

If you decide to take probiotics, make sure that prebiotics are mixed into them. The food industry started to "fortify" their products with prebiotics which will show up in the list of ingredients as Galactooligosaccharide (GOS), Fructooligosaccharide (FOS), Oligofructose, or just inulin. The first two prebiotics seems to enhance the growth of bifidobacterial and lactobacilli. GOS, for instance, is produced in the body. 90% of the fiber in women's breast milk is, in fact, GOS. Babies that are bottle-fed with formula milk benefit from added GOS. Screenings of their gut bacteria showed a similarly diverse gut microbiome to that of breastfed babies. Further, studies show that babies that are only fed formula milk without GOS are more prone to develop allergies and neurodermatitis. GOS takes on another important role in the gut: it takes away space from bad gut bacteria by docking on to the gut cells that are otherwise favored locations of pathogens.[122]

Lesson 28

We don't sit correctly on the toilet

No one really wants to talk about what happens when they withdraw to the restroom. But when you hear that a common place of death in older, unathletic people is right there, it does make you wonder what the cause might be.

It turns out the sitting position Western cultures have adopted ever since the invention of toilets is the problem. Commonly, when seated on a toilet the legs will be in a 90-degree or bigger-angled position with a pretty straight back. The way the closure mechanism of the gut is designed, though, it does not open in this position. There is a kink in the tube leading to the exit. The muscle that encircles the gut is strapped around it like a lasso when seated. The only way to straighten the tube and loosen the lasso is by squatting – the natural defecation position of humans since the beginning of time.

People that are not aware of these mechanisms, tend to tense up, even to the extent that their abdominal muscles are flexed, on the toilet when trying to push out the stool. This leads to a build-up of pressure. Healthy, young adults might get away with it but anyone not so lucky can experience hemorrhoids as a consequence. The worst case is an older, unathletic person suffering from arteriosclerosis trying to push too hard. The hatch is tightly closed, leading to pressure travelling up the body causing an artery to burst – boom, death by stroke in the restroom! This can be avoided by slightly bending forward and positioning a little chair, also referred to as "squatty potty" in conventional stores, under your feet.

Roman has the squatty potty readily available in every room for his guests during the fast.

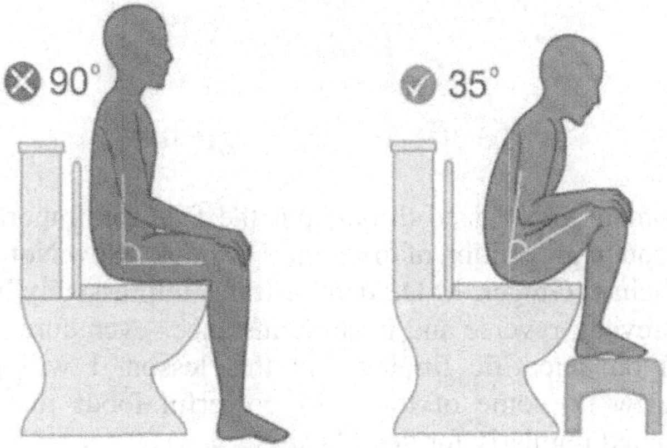

***Figure 3:** Incorrect vs. correct sitting position*

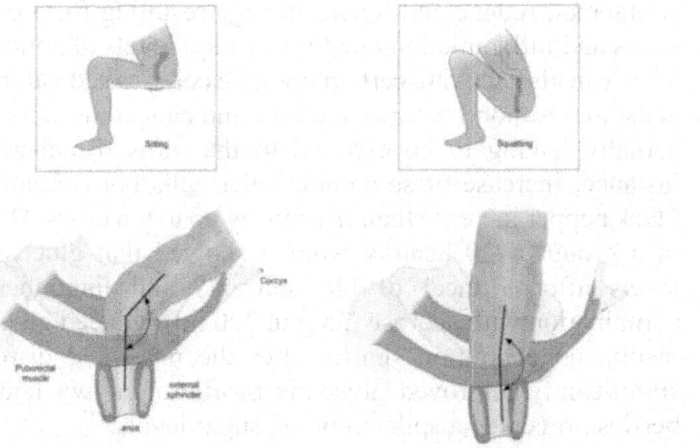

***Figure 4:** Left illustration shows kink in gut when sitting; right illustration shows straight gut when squatting*

Lesson 29

Foods to eat regularly

Roman emphasized throughout the fast, the importance of nutrition in prevention of diseases. The book "How Not To Die" by Michael Greger, M.D., demonstrates impressively how diet can prevent, reverse and in some instances even cure illnesses based on scientific findings. In this lesson, I will give an overview on some of the most powerful foods that can be consumed regularly for good health.

Fruits that should be eaten on a daily basis are berries. They counteract, reduce and repair damage resulting from oxidative stress and inflammation due to their high levels of antioxidants. They can also activate certain immune cells, called natural killer cells, that respond to virus-infected and cancerous cells without actually having to be exposed to the virus. Blueberries, for instance, increase these natural killer cells but cardamom and black pepper increase their *activity* by up to ten times. One study in a group of 20 healthy women showed that glucose blood levels after a meal of blackcurrants and lingonberries in combination with sucrose (35 g in 300 ml) reduced glucose and insulin concentration shortly after the meal and displayed a significantly improved glycemic profile after two hours. The berries prevented a spike in blood sugar levels.[123]

If there are vegetables that can be recommended to consume daily, it is the group of cruciferous vegetables. This group contains such produce as arugula, bok choy, broccoli, brussels sprouts, cabbage (white and red, the latter being especially rich in antioxidants), cauliflower, collard greens, radishes, kale, kohlrabi, mustard, horseradish, turnips, wasabi and watercress, to list a few. They have shown to be potent in preventing DNA damage and metastatic cancer spread, boost liver detoxication, reduce the risk of prostate cancer progression and can help the body's immune system in fighting pathogens and pollutants. Many of the health benefits can be attributed to sulforaphane, a compound found predominantly in cruciferous vegetables. It has shown to be effective in treating prostate cancer, asthma, lung diseases such as COPD (chronic obstructive pulmonary disease), and even autism. It seems to protect the brain against neurodegenerative diseases, the eyes against oxidative stress and attenuates nasal allergic response to diesel exhaust particles. Raw broccoli, brussels sprouts and cauliflower work especially well in suppressing cancer growth. A precursor is needed to react with the enzyme in the vegetable to form sulforaphane in a first step. However, the enzyme is deactivated when the vegetables are cooked. Keep in mind, that heat does not affect the precursor. One way to activate the chemical reaction that triggers the formation of sulforaphane is to chop, chew or otherwise damage the cruciferous vegetable. After 40 minutes all the sulforaphane is produced and the veggies can be safely cooked. Alternatively, you can buy pre-chopped or shredded cruciferous vegetables. When you buy frozen broccoli, however, the manufacturer normally flash-cooks the vegetable. In order to activate the dead enzyme, there is an easy trick: mustard powder. Mustard seeds contain the enzyme that can react with cruciferous vegetables. Sprinkle mustard powder on frozen broccoli, and sulforaphane will be produced.

Another group of vegetables with the most cancer-preventing potential are allium vegetables, such as garlic, onion, chives, leek, scallion and shallot. They seem to be particularly powerful when it comes to the protection against cancers of the gastrointestinal tract. Studies have shown that mechanisms are in place that reduce the activation of carcinogens.[124] Allicin, the defense molecule present in allium vegetables, in particular raw garlic, has a broad antimicrobial spectrum to defend even against antibiotic resistant strains and fungi.[125]

One tablespoon of ground flaxseeds can be recommended to eat daily. Avoid whole flaxseeds, since the grain is sharp and might injure the inside of your intestines, plus, unless they are fully chewed, no nutrients will be released. Make sure to drink enough water with the flaxseeds as they extract water and bulk up in the stomach. It is easy to add it to smoothies, oatmeal or salads. Alternatively, it can be used as an egg substitute. One tablespoon of flaxseeds mixed with three tablespoons of water will make for a gooey substance that can be used as a binding agent in baked goods.[126] Flaxseeds help reduce high blood pressure, lower bad cholesterol, help control triglyceride, as well as, help in fighting breast and prostate cancer, regulate blood sugar, reduce inflammation and treat constipation due to its laxative effect. It is the content of alpha-linolenic acid, omega-3 fatty acids, the array of antioxidants, lignans, and fiber that give the seed its power in supporting human health.[127] Lignans are phytoestrogens that are common in the plant kingdom but stand out in flaxseeds where they are up to 100 times more present. Lignans can diminish estrogen's potentially negative effects and are used as such in medical therapy for menstrual breast pain. Regular consumption can prevent breast cancer by prolonging the menstrual cycle of a woman by one day. As a result, the woman will have fewer periods throughout her life and thus, less estrogen exposure that can lead to breast cancer.[128]

Whole grains, like barley, buckwheat, bulgur, oats, brown rice, millet, popcorn, quinoa, rye, whole wheat pasta and wild rice, have been found to be very beneficial. One meta study that was conducted in 2015 concluded that life expectancy significantly increases in people who eat more whole grains.[129] Whole grains are associated with lower risk of major chronic diseases, like type 2 diabetes and cardiovascular diseases. The fiber and other nutrients, such as B vitamins, iron, folate, selenium, potassium and magnesium contribute to the coverage of some basic vitamins and trace minerals. Many studies attest to the inflammation-lowering properties of a whole grain-based diet. The fiber and phytochemicals in whole grains positively influence how the microbiome transforms certain bioactive substances to moderate low-grade inflammation. Treat yourself to three servings every day!

Legumes are another group of foods I can highly recommend to add to your daily meals. A study in 2012 showed that regular consumption of pulses (beans, peas and lentils) reduced the risk of developing metabolic syndrome in overweight and obese adults. One group was advised to reduce their caloric intake by 500 calories per day, while the other group had to include five cups of pulses per week ad libitum over eight weeks. The subjects allowed to eat more were as effective at improving markers for metabolic syndrome as the group instructed to eat less. The pulse group, however, improved their insulin regulation and increased the good cholesterol. The researchers did consider the possibility of the pulse-eaters eating less other unhealthy foods – after all, legumes are extremely filling.[130] Often times when you try to add certain food groups in certain amounts, a natural side effect will be the lack of capacity to eat other empty calories. If you ask me, that's a win-win situation!

Herbs and spices have become one of my favorite additions to both, savory and sweet meals, as well as drinks. Feel free to experiment and add dried or fresh basil, cilantro, dill, oregano, marjoram, rosemary or thyme to your dishes. Many flavorful spices more commonly used in curries that can be added are chili powder, cumin, coriander seeds, ginger, paprika (smoked or regular) and cayenne pepper. Lately I spice up my coffees with a combination of allspice, cinnamon, cloves, cardamom and nutmeg.

Have you ever wondered what makes aspirin the most commonly used drug in the world? Its active ingredient is salicylic acid. Aspirin is taken by millions of people daily as a blood thinner to prevent strokes. Further, it is known for its anti-inflammatory properties. Salicylic acid, though, is a compound that can naturally be found in plants, fruits and vegetables. Herbs and spices contain the highest concentrations of salicylic acid. While cardamom, tamarind and turmeric are rich in the compound, cumin has the biggest natural occurrence of salicylic acid. One teaspoon of ground cumin has equivalent amounts of the lower-dosed, so-called baby aspirin.[131] Cumin and ground coriander seeds are the main spices of falafel – I make them regularly in my air fryer with tons of fresh parsley and cilantro. Turmeric is one of the spices I can recommend to eat daily. I add it in my tea with matcha powder and black pepper. Thousands of studies came out over the last years, researching curcumin, one of the potent compounds that gives turmeric its bright, yellow color. The findings overlap: curcumin is anti-inflammatory, anti-carcinogenic, anti-bacterial, anti-fungal, pulmonary-protective, cardio- and liver-protective, an antioxidant, neuro-protective, insulin-sensitizing and thrombo-suppressive. It effectively treats osteoarthritis, rheumatoid arthritis, lupus, inflammatory bowel disease, as well as protects against various cancers and speeds up recovery after surgery.[132] In India, the spice is consumed frequently as an ingredient in curries, thus, the daily recommendation is based on their average intake: one quarter teaspoon. In order to get the most benefits from turmeric, combine it with black pepper. A compound in black pepper inhibits drug metabolism. An hour after eating turmeric, only small trace amounts of curcumin circulate in the blood stream. Your liver is filtering out the foreign substance. By combining turmeric with a quarter teaspoon of black pepper, curcumin levels in your blood shoots up by 2,000 percent. Realistically you will not add that much black pepper but luckily even a tiny amount of black pepper will boost curcumin in your blood. Adding a source of fat can even further enhance the bioavailability of curcumin by seven to eight times.[133]

This lesson wouldn't be complete if I didn't include nuts. Eat nuts every day, ideally one serving (2 tablespoons of nut or seed butter or ¼ cup nuts or seeds). Nuts protect from cardiovascular diseases by regulating cholesterol levels. They also protect from weight gain, in some instances even help in weight loss. A 2012 study of Chinese subjects with metabolic syndrome impressively demonstrated the weight control properties of nuts.

Individuals ate up to 70 g of pistachios (or around 122 pistachios if the average pistachio with its shell weighs 0.57 g) as a snack on a daily basis for three months. They did not gain weight. Is removing the shells helpful maybe in slowing down consumption and thus, you feel full quicker? Or is it all the chewing? Could it be that parts of the nut aren't digested and leave your body undigested again? 70% of nut calories are lost through dietary compensation, 10% leave the body as fat through your stool. The remaining 20% are sped up metabolism that burns your own fat. Walnuts stand out by burning 31 g of fat versus 20 g of fat burning in subjects eating the same number of calories and fat from other sources. The omega-3 fatty acids are particularly high in walnuts, making them exceptionally beneficial.[134]

Certain fruits, vegetables, spices and nuts have been highlighted here but please keep in mind that variety is still key. As much as one nut or spice might stand out with its health benefits, at the end of the day your gut microbiome and body need a wide variety of nutrients and foods to function properly.

Lesson 30

Don't go grocery shopping hungry

Towards the end of the fast, Roman started to prepare us for our return home; and with that, being responsible for preparing our own meals and doing our shopping.

A supermarket is set up in a way that will tempt you to impulse purchases. You will see "deals", "special offers", "lower price" and "sale" signs throughout the shop. Many of the offerings are processed snacks, candy and soft drinks. Once you think that you are done and ready to check out, you approach the cashier. There is a line. You have to wait. You are tired from reading all the ingredient lists (hopefully!), your willpower is lessened and you see this one treat that you really like: next thing you know you check out snack XYZ. Supermarkets strategically place these items near the registry. Manufacturers pay, in fact, extra to get these prime locations. Similar mechanisms are at work with items placed at eye-level; they are more expensive than bottom-shelf products. Grocery stores also tap into your sense of smell and, thus, into your hunger. The baked goods, the deliciously smelling deli meats, maybe a rotisserie chicken. The entire supermarket is set-up in a way where most basic and often bought items are spread out so that customers have to pass certain "tempting" aisles they would normally avoid.

To avoid buying unnecessary items, prepare a shopping list before you go shopping. Only items that make it home, can be devoured in a weak moment. Remove the temptation of unhealthy snacks, by removing the choice at home. Do not go shopping hungry. You do not lack self-discipline when you are hungry and end up buying something you didn't need. It is almost impossible to work against your body's self-preservation mode where your brain will "reason" you into buying junk. But with the understanding that you can't "out-reason" a hungry brain, you can try to out-smart it by going prepared, sticking to your shopping list and making sure you are not hungry. Also keep in mind that you can fall victim to "decision fatigue", a phenomenon that explains humans' limited capacity to make many decisions in a short period of time, and the quality of these decisions deteriorating up to the point where irrational choices are made. All your self-resolve will wear you down after a while, if you are not used to certain shopping habits.

Disclaimer: The following lesson is meant for educational purpose only. It should not replace treatment from a medical professional. Before following any advice, the reader is encouraged to conduct their own research in partnership with a health care professional.

Lesson 31

H_2O_2 cure

Have you heard of hyperbaric oxygen therapy (HBOT)? HBOT is a therapy where subjects are placed in a pressure chamber breathing 100% oxygen. HBOT is one type of oxygen therapy that has been around since the 1950s. The aim is to increase oxygen in the body and thus, allow it to heal itself. In 2020 researchers in Israel used HBOT in healthy 64+ year old adults and impressively demonstrated age-reversing effects: they increased telomere length which normally shortens with age, improved cognitive functions and boosted natural killer and B cells (both crucial in immune responses). The increased oxygen levels in the blood release growth hormones and stem cells that promote healing.[135] And all simply by enriching blood with oxygen! The costs vary from $250 to $450 per treatment, depending on location and services. What if I told you, you can have the same effect for a couple of cents?

Roman does a hydrogen peroxide cure each year for two months where he orally ingests 3% H_2O_2 diluted in water. He uses it to reduce his genetically high cholesterol levels but it also kills any bacteria, viruses, fungi, yeast and other organisms that have no business in your body. He advises to gradually build up to 10 drops three times a day.

	Morning	Lunch	Dinner
Day 1	1 drop	1 drop	1 drop
Day 2	2 drops	2 drops	2 drops
Day 3	3 drops	3 drops	3 drops
...			
...			
Day 9	9 drops	9 drops	9 drops
Day 1 of the 2-month H_2O_2 cure	10 drops	10 drops	10 drops

Since this book is aimed at an American audience, I will present the hydrogen peroxide cure as described in *The one-minute cure: the secret of healing virtually all diseases* by Madison Cavanaugh. According to the author the number of drops should be diluted in 6 to 8 ounces distilled water. Do not use tap water; it contains chloride and can react with the hydrogen peroxide.

	Morning	Lunch	Dinner
Day 1	3 drops	3 drops	3 drops
Day 2	4 drops	4 drops	4 drops
Day 3	5 drops	5 drops	5 drops
Day 4	6 drops	6 drops	6 drops
Day 5	7 drops	7 drops	7 drops
Day 6	8 drops	8 drops	8 drops
Day 7	9 drops	9 drops	9 drops
Day 8	10 drops	10 drops	10 drops
Day 9	11 drops	11 drops	11 drops
Day 10	12 drops	12 drops	12 drops
Day 11	13 drops	13 drops	13 drops

Day 12	14 drops	14 drops	14 drops
Day 13	15 drops	15 drops	15 drops
Day 14	16 drops	16 drops	16 drops
Day 15	17 drops	17 drops	17 drops
Day 16	18 drops	18 drops	18 drops
Day 17	19 drops	19 drops	19 drops
Day 18	20 drops	20 drops	20 drops
Day 19	21 drops	21 drops	21 drops
Day 20	22 drops	22 drops	22 drops
Day 21	23 drops	23 drops	23 drops
Day 22	24 drops	24 drops	24 drops
Day 23	**25 drops**	**25 drops**	**25 drops**
Day 24	24 drops	24 drops	24 drops
Day 25	23 drops	23 drops	23 drops
Day 26	22 drops	22 drops	22 drops
Day 27	21 drops	21 drops	21 drops
Day 28	20 drops	20 drops	20 drops
Day 29	19 drops	19 drops	19 drops
Day 30	18 drops	18 drops	18 drops
Day 31	17 drops	17 drops	17 drops
Day 32	16 drops	16 drops	16 drops
Day 33	15 drops	15 drops	15 drops
Day 34	14 drops	14 drops	14 drops
Day 35	13 drops	13 drops	13 drops
Day 36	12 drops	12 drops	12 drops
Day 37	11 drops	11 drops	11 drops
Day 38	10 drops	10 drops	10 drops
Day 39	9 drops	9 drops	9 drops

Day 40	8 drops	8 drops	8 drops
Day 41	7 drops	7 drops	7 drops
Day 42	6 drops	6 drops	6 drops
Day 43	5 drops	5 drops	5 drops
Day 44	4 drops	4 drops	4 drops
Day 45	3 drops	3 drops	3 drops

After 23 days, the intake is reduced by one drop each day until the maintenance level of 3 drops is reached. In total, this cure will take a little less than 1.5 months. Cavanaugh bases the regiment on many years of experience and reported success by thousands of users. It seems like Cavanaugh suggests to continue taking the 3 drops daily, and even offers for more serious conditions to try taking 25 drops three times a day for one to three weeks during the beginning of the maintenance phase, then reduce 25 drops to taking only twice a day for up to six months. Alternatively, the maintenance schedule can be adjusted to taking 5 to 15 drops based on how a person feels. Listen to your body: one woman reported that from taking 20 drops her skin became too dry; she reduced the intake.

Important to notice is that H_2O_2 needs to be taken on an empty stomach since the reaction with fatty acids produces hydroxyl radicals which can harm the lining of the intestines. Take it at least one hour before a meal and/or at least three hours after mealtime. Only food-grade peroxide diluted in distilled water is safe for internal use. Regular 3% pharmaceutical grade or other peroxides contain stabilizers such as acetanilide, phenol, sodium stagnate and tetrasodium phosphate.[136] In the US only 35% food-grade H_2O_2 can be used. In Germany, for instance, it is possible to purchase a 3% food-grade peroxide.[137] The 35% grade needs to be diluted, otherwise it can cause severe damage to your body. It helps to pour the peroxide into a small glass bottle with an eyedropper cap. The remaining bottle can be kept in the fridge or freezer. Label your bottle "35% Food

Grade Hydrogen Peroxide". There was one story about a person not realizing that the 35% grade cannot be swallowed as is, due to the fact that it contains the word "food" in it, thinking it is safe for ingestion. If you want to make sure no one in your household drinks it, label it differently (draw a skull on the bottle or add the word *toxic* for example). Few people reported to feel nauseas, fatigued or experienced diarrhea and cold-like symptoms. These symptoms are linked to your body working hard in ridding itself of toxins. It is important to continue the therapy.[138]

H_2O_2 helps the body rid itself of viruses, harmful bacteria, toxins and pathogens. Cavanaugh lists an extensive array of diseases and ailments that can be treated with bio-oxidative therapy:

AIDS	Cystitis	Lupus Erythematosis
Acne	Diabetes Type II	Lymphoma
Allergies	Diabetic Gangrene	Metastatic Carcinoma
Altitude Sickness	Diabetic Retinopathy	Migraine headaches
Alzheimer's Disease	Digestion Problems	Mononucleosis
Anemia	Eczema	Multiple Sclerosis
Angina	Emphysema	Open sores and wounds
Arrhythmia	Epstein-Barr infection	Parasitic infections
Arteriosclerosis	Food allergies	Parkinson's Disease
Arthritis	Fungal infections	Periodontal Disease
Asthma	Fungus	Proctitis
Bacterial Infections	Gangrene	Prostatitis
Bronchitis	Gingivitis	Rheumatoid Arthritis

Burns	Gum Disease	Shingles
Cancer	Headaches	Sinusitis
Candidiasis	Hepatitis	Sore Throat
Cardiovascular Disease	Herpes	Temporal Arteritis
Cerebral Vascular Disease	Herpes Simplex	Trichomoniasis
Cholesterol (High)	Herpes Zoster	Ulcers
Chronic Pain	HIV Infection	Vascular Diseases
Cirrhosis of the liver	Influenza	Vascular headaches
Cluster headaches	Insect bites	Viral infections
Colitis	Leg ulcers	Warts
COPD	Leukemia	Yeast infection

People who underwent an organ transplant should not use any hydrogen peroxide cures. While hydrogen peroxide increases the activity of your immune system, people who received an organ need to suppress immune activity to ensure that the organ is not rejected by their body.

Let's take a look at the science behind. Hydrogen peroxide is a byproduct of many common metabolic processes in our body and can be damaging to important proteins and DNA if not broken down by the body immediately. That's where catalase comes into play. Catalase is a powerful enzyme that converts hydrogen peroxide to water and oxygen. A single molecule can convert millions of hydrogen peroxide molecules into water and oxygen each second. This way catalase can protect the cell from oxidative damage. Catalase is present in almost all creatures that can survive and grow in an oxygenated environment, so-called aerobic organisms. Anaerobic organisms, on the other hand, might not require oxygen to live and may even die in the presence of it.

In 1931 Dr. Otto Warburg made an important discovery that was awarded with the Nobel Prize in Physiology or Medicine: he proved that viruses cannot proliferate or exist in aerobic or oxygen-rich environments. Ninety years ago, Dr. Warburg stated as the primary cause of cancer the insufficient amounts of oxygen on a cellular level and therefore, inferred from it that cancer cells couldn't survive in an aerobic environment. This was proven time and again in various studies. While unwanted organisms are eliminated under high oxygen levels, healthy cells thrive and become more resilient.[139]

Catalase is abundant in humans, in particular in our plasma and red cells. Hydrogen peroxide reacts in a first instance with catalase in the plasma and white blood cells. Once it penetrates the cell wall of red blood cells, it reacts with the existing catalase within the cell, leading to the release of additional oxygen – the blood becomes supersaturated with oxygen, also called hyperoxia. In addition, the peroxide disassociates oxygen and hemoglobin, leading to maximized delivery of oxygen from the blood to the cells. More importantly, though, your white blood cells produce H_2O_2 when they detect an invading organism that needs to be neutralized. Hydrogen peroxide further stimulates the production of interferon, a protein produced when the presence of viruses is detected. Most bacteria, fungi, yeast, parasites and viruses respond well to hydrogen peroxide and can be killed off because they either have no catalase or only very little.[140] This would explain how good bacteria are not affected by H_2O_2; they are aerobic organisms and thrive in an oxygenated atmosphere.

Japanese researchers presented in 2007 their findings in the treatment of chemotherapy-resistant tumors of the skin with hydrogen peroxide solution. They discovered that after the treatment with the peroxide, the tumor cells became sensitive to the radiation and could be killed. The method was named Kochi Oxydol-Radiation Therapy for Unresectable Carcinomas (KORTUC I). In 2009 KORTUC II was developed for patients with recurrent breast cancer. The therapy is done by injecting hydrogen peroxide and the salt of hyaluronic acid into the tumor, followed by radiation therapy. Over the course of treatments, the cancers were successfully treated and patients were left tumor-free, with few side effects that subsided quickly. With this type of therapy, surgery was avoided.[141]

There are many counterclaims on the usefulness of hydrogen peroxide, one of such a study from 2011. It seemed to show that cancer cells can thrive both, in aerobic and anaerobic environments and even secrete hydrogen peroxide, prompting the belief that tumors can actually grow in the presence of peroxide.[142]

A study in 2016 has shown that intravenous injections of large vitamin C (ascorbic acid) amounts create hydrogen peroxide. The concentration is 100 to 500 times higher in the blood when vitamin C is injected intravenous versus taking vitamin C orally due to the bypassing of normal gut metabolism and excretion pathways. The study showed that tumor cells have a decreased ability to metabolize hydrogen peroxide, contrary to normal cells that have the ability to remove H_2O_2. The researchers were able to demonstrate the toxicity of H_2O_2 to cancer cells.[143]

Other natural sources of hydrogen peroxide are breast milk and coffee. Breast milk plays an important role in the development of a child's immune system. Part of it is due to its hydrogen peroxide content that stimulates the baby's immune response and the activation of metabolic processes. Coffee was found to be another source of naturally occurring hydrogen peroxide source. When consumed in the conventional manner, it contains hydrogen peroxide of approximately 750 micrograms. Let it sit longer and the peroxide production will increase up to 24 hours.[144] Does that sound familiar? Cold brew coffee is one drink trending in recent years with its proclaimed health benefits. Could it be the hydrogen peroxide content that makes it so powerful?

The successful treatment of diseases with hydrogen peroxide goes back to India during World War I where intravenous injections in critically sick soldiers with pneumonia were treated. Dr. T.H. Oliver was able to cut the mortality rate from 80% to 48% in 25 patients that were deemed terminally ill – 13 soldiers recovered. Much of the scientific benefits of hydrogen peroxide stem from intravenous therapies performed by trained physicians. One common concern of intravenous administration, was the occurrence of gas embolism. Physicians saw high success rates when the hydrogen peroxide solution was administered slowly with sufficient breaks so that the oxygen could be absorbed immediately.[145]

Especially effective was the treatment on people suffering from emphysema, a lung disease most commonly seen in smokers and people exposed to industrial pollutants characterized by damage to the walls of the air sacs. Symptoms are reduced lung capacity and a persistent cough. The heart has to work harder to circulate blood and heart failure ends up being often the cause of death. Hydrogen peroxide has shown to improve breathing when used in a vaporizer or humidifier (one ounce of 35% food-grade H_2O_2 in a gallon of water) over night. Even better results have been achieved when the peroxide was injected intravenously. The mucus is loosened in the lining of the lungs by the added oxygen and propelled out of the lungs through coughing. Many success stories have been reported from emphysema sufferers trying this approach.[146]

It seems like general acceptance of hydrogen peroxide use was experienced in the 60s of Europe where physicians in Germany and Russia prescribed peroxide commonly. Other bio-oxidative therapies involving ozone (O3) had been used in Germany to treat and even cure AIDS patients. Most prominently among them is Dr. Alexander Preuss who publicized his findings on ozone therapy that he claims saved the lives of at least ten people suffering from AIDS. Many more case studies exist from the 1980s in the US where patients suffering from chronic fatigue syndrome – often times either caused by Epstein-Barr virus or candida – or multiple sclerosis were successfully treated with H_2O_2. Further, ointments made with 10% to 20% hydrogen peroxide have been tremendously successful in treating blood flow disorders in pregnant women and diabetics, as well as treating warts. The skin seems to be great at absorbing the peroxide and quickly passing it on to deep tissue where it lasts for a long time. A future application of the balm is only required two or three days later. Absorption through the skin is in fact so great, that people have reported to bathe in it, using 1 to 8 pints (1 pint = 0.4732 liters) of 3% solution to a tub full of warm water, feeling awake and energized after the oxygen boost.[147]

But why do these stories not make headlines? One explanation is that H_2O_2 could be the death of the trillion-dollar pharma industry. The peroxide is not patentable and dirt cheap to purchase. All I could find on the topic are case studies; no large-scale research has been ever conducted on oral ingestion or intravenous injections of hydrogen peroxide. Who would want to fund that anyways?

I personally tried Roman's therapy of two months and ten days. He recommends to up the dosage to 20 drops three times a day when hit with a disease like a cold or flu for the duration of the symptoms. Once you don't have any symptoms, you stop the intake. You could even use a nasal spray. Fill it with a diluted 3% hydrogen peroxide solution, pump it five to ten times into your mouth while inhaling deeply the mist. Follow this regiment twice in the morning and twice at night. If you are battling a respiratory disease, use the spray every two hours.

Both, my husband and I, contracted coronavirus this year. While he opted for conventional medication, I took hydrogen peroxide. Prior to the infection, we were exercising regularly, eating well and taking probiotics. Neither one of has had an underlying medical condition. My symptoms were more mild and shorter than his. Neither one of us developed lasting damage from the infection. Of course, I can't know if there is a causal relationship between my milder symptoms and taking the hydrogen peroxide or other health choices I made around that time. After all, that year I had gone on my second 10-day fast – my husband didn't – I ate extremely clean, incorporating Roman's suggestion for 600 g of vegetables, 400 g of fruits daily and most days 100 g of legumes, plus I worked out regularly in the harsh winter of Vienna. Could those have been the determining factors? We won't know. All we know, is that many good decisions probably will lead to good overall health.

Another contributing factor not many people talk about when it comes to healing, is the role stress plays in the operation of your cells. It is one thing to enrich your blood with oxygen but another one for your cells to actually receive that oxygen. Under normal circumstance, when everything is calm in your life, your body will operate on the parasympathetic nervous system. You will be able to digest food, extract nutrients and run all your organs properly. That's because your cells are open. They are able to receive oxygen, absorb nutrients and expel waste products. A hydrogen peroxide cure will be under such circumstances successful due to the cells' ability to take in the oxygen. But what happens when you experience stress? That can be from an actual life-threatening situation to emotional stress experienced due to fear, anxiety, concern or worry. That is when your sympathetic nervous system takes over. It will prepare you for fight-or-flight by moving your blood away from digestion and into your muscles, glucose is released back into the bloodstream and your heart rate is increased with the help of adrenaline. You are revved up and ready to go. Unfortunately, most people nowadays don't only stay temporarily in this state but are trapped in a lifestyle of one stressful situation after another. On a cellular level, your cells shut down, and with that nutrition absorption is halted, as well as oxygen receipt. You are starving your cells of the one thing that keeps them alive. If a cell stays oxygen deprived long enough, it becomes cancerous. Many ancient practices like yoga, Qi Gong and meditation in their essence preach the importance of breathing and with it underline the role oxygen plays in the human body. Even Wim Hof's practice of cold exposure is in its core a way to enrich your blood with oxygen which in turn will lower your inflammation and potentially heal you.[148]

Lesson 32

Why you should fast for 36 hours every week

Fasting for 36 hours every week will give you the following benefits:

Weight management

- to maintain your current weight; allows for the occasional cheat meal without necessarliy putting on weight

Reset taste buds

- the break allows for less usage of sugar and salt after the fast without necessarily compromising on satisfaction from meal

Lowered inflammations

- the body has time to focus on healing while not burdened with digestion

Anti-ageing properties

- by getting into a state of authophagy the body can dispose of accumulated cell damage and rid itself of oxidative stress

Better sleep

- longer time is spent in REM phase, which is crucial for memory retantion and overall mental health and well-being
- wake up better rested and focused the next day

Cleaning of intestines

- intestines can only clean themselves when they have long enough breaks from digesting food

After dinner on Sunday night, I fast for at least 36 hours until breakfast on Tuesday morning. Whether you believe it or not, I look forward to it every week! Initially, when I returned from the fasts, I did not feel like I could commit to fasting once a week, especially while working. The major problem was that I underate and restricted myself continuously. Once I started to eat as much as I wanted by listening to my body, I realized I needed a break from all the feasting. All of a sudden, it wasn't difficult anymore to abstain from food for one day. To me, Monday is the perfect day for a fast. Most times I enjoy my cheat meals on the weekends when going on my social outings. It is easy not to schedule any outings at the beginning of the week, even though, I have reached a point where I don't even mind people eating around me while I fast.

If this is too extreme for you, a better approach could be to start off with 12-hour fasts. From there you can attempt 14, then 16 then 18 hours.

Whichever approach you choose, I wish you success in you endeavors to a healthier, better life!

ENDNOTES

[1] Alexey Kokosov and Sergey Osinin, *Therapeutic Fasting (RDT) for Bronchial Asthma* (Tashkent: Siberika Publishing, 1984).

[2] Sylvie Gilman and Thierry de Lestrade, "Fasten und Heilen – Altes Wissen und neueste Forschung," Documentary, March 29, 2012.

[3] "Fasting," Encyclopedia, *Encyclopedia Britannica* (blog), accessed June 3, 2021, https://www.britannica.com/topic/fasting.

[4] University of East Anglia, "How Fasting Diets Could Harm Future Generations," *ScienceDaily*, May 11, 2021, www.sciencedaily.com/releases/2021/05/210511201128.htm.

[5] "Fasting."

[6] Soutik Biswas, "Should India's Jains Be given the Choice to Die?," *BBC News*, August 21, 2015, https://www.bbc.com/news/world-asia-india-33998688.

[7] "Fasting."

[8] "The Nobel Prize in Physiology or Medicine 2016," Press release (NobelPrize.org, October 3, 2016), https://www.nobelprize.org/prizes/medicine/2016/press-release/.

[9] "Heiße Quellen Am Baikalsee [Heilende Wirkungen & Beste Orte]," *Russland Erleben* (blog), accessed June 9, 2021, https://www.russland-erleben.com/baikalsee-heisse-quellen/.

[10] Gilman and de Lestrade, "Fasten und Heilen – Altes Wissen und neueste Forschung."

[11] Kokosov and Osinin, *Therapeutic Fasting (RDT) for Bronchial Asthma.*

[12] Gilman and de Lestrade, "Fasten und Heilen – Altes Wissen und neueste Forschung."

[13] "Fastenkrise – Und Nun?," March 18, 2020, https://www.fitreisen.de/blog/fastenkrise-und-nun/.

[14] Gilman and de Lestrade, "Fasten und Heilen – Altes Wissen und neueste Forschung."

[15] "Fastenkrise – Und Nun?"

[16] Gilman and de Lestrade, "Fasten und Heilen – Altes Wissen und neueste Forschung."

[17] "Fastenkrise – Und Nun?"

[18] Y Le Maho, J-P Robin, and Y Cherel, "Starvation as a Treatment of Obesity: The Need to Conserve Body Protein," *Physiology* 3, no. 1

(February 1, 1988): 21–24, https://doi.org/10.1152/physiologyonline.1988.3.1.21.

[19] Gilman and de Lestrade, "Fasten und Heilen – Altes Wissen und neueste Forschung."

[20] Gilman and de Lestrade.

[21] Kokosov and Osinin, *Therapeutic Fasting (RDT) for Bronchial Asthma*.

[22] Gilman and de Lestrade, "Fasten und Heilen – Altes Wissen und neueste Forschung."

[23] Gilman and de Lestrade.

[24] "Neue Formen Des Fastens," *Domradio* (blog), June 10, 2020, https://www.domradio.de/themen/glaube/2020-06-10/neue-formen-des-fastens-studie-viele-menschen-haben-schon-einmal-gefastet.

[25] Klinik Dr. Otto Buchinger GmbH & Co. KG, "Buchinger," n.d., accessed June 20, 2021.

[26] Gilman and de Lestrade, "Fasten und Heilen – Altes Wissen und neueste Forschung."

[27] P. R. Kerndt et al., "Fasting: The History, Pathophysiology and Complications," *The Western Journal of Medicine* 137, no. 5 (November 1982): 379–99.

[28] Dr. Jason Fung, *The Obesity Code: Unlocking the Secrets of Weight Loss* (Carlton North: Scribe Publications, 2016).

[29] John Jaquish and Henry Alkire, *Weight Lifting Is a Waste of Time: So Is Cardio, and There's a Better Way to Have the Body You Want*, 2020.

[30] Gilman and de Lestrade, "Fasten und Heilen – Altes Wissen und neueste Forschung."

[31] Rainer Stange and Claus Leitzmann, eds., *Ernährung und Fasten als Therapie*, 2., vollständig aktualisierte Auflage, Naturheilverfahren (Berlin; [Heidelberg]: Springer, 2018).

[32] Gilman and de Lestrade, "Fasten und Heilen – Altes Wissen und neueste Forschung."

[33] Francesco Plotti et al., "Diet and Chemotherapy: The Effects of Fasting and Ketogenic Diet on Cancer Treatment," *Chemotherapy* 65, no. 3–4 (2020): 77–84, https://doi.org/10.1159/000510839.

[34] Stefanie de Groot et al., "The Effects of Short-Term Fasting on Tolerance to (Neo) Adjuvant Chemotherapy in HER2-Negative Breast Cancer Patients: A Randomized Pilot Study," *BMC Cancer* 15, no. 1 (December 2015): 652, https://doi.org/10.1186/s12885-015-1663-5.

[35] Tanya B. Dorff et al., "Safety and Feasibility of Fasting in Combination with Platinum-Based Chemotherapy," *BMC Cancer* 16, no. 1 (December 2016): 360, https://doi.org/10.1186/s12885-016-2370-6.

[36] Stephan P. Bauersfeld et al., "The Effects of Short-Term Fasting on Quality of Life and Tolerance to Chemotherapy in Patients with Breast and Ovarian Cancer: A Randomized Cross-over Pilot Study," *BMC Cancer* 18, no. 1 (December 2018): 476, https://doi.org/10.1186/s12885-018-4353-2.

[37] Gilman and de Lestrade, "Fasten und Heilen – Altes Wissen und neueste Forschung."

[38] Chia-Wei Cheng et al., "Prolonged Fasting Reduces IGF-1/PKA to Promote Hematopoietic-Stem-Cell-Based Regeneration and Reverse Immunosuppression," *Cell Stem Cell* 14, no. 6 (June 2014): 810–23, https://doi.org/10.1016/j.stem.2014.04.014.

[39] Roman Fessler, "Heilfasteninstitut Fessler," accessed June 9, 2021, https://www.heilfasten.at/.

[40] Fung, *The Obesity Code.*

[41] Leah M. Kalm and Richard D. Semba, "They Starved So That Others Be Better Fed: Remembering Ancel Keys and the Minnesota Experiment," *The Journal of Nutrition* 135, no. 6 (June 1, 2005): 1347–52, https://doi.org/10.1093/jn/135.6.1347.

[42] Michael Rosenbaum et al., "Long-Term Persistence of Adaptive Thermogenesis in Subjects Who Have Maintained a Reduced Body Weight," *The American Journal of Clinical Nutrition* 88, no. 4 (October 1, 2008): 906–12, https://doi.org/10.1093/ajcn/88.4.906.

[43] Priya Sumithran et al., "Long-Term Persistence of Hormonal Adaptations to Weight Loss," *New England Journal of Medicine* 365, no. 17 (October 27, 2011): 1597–1604, https://doi.org/10.1056/NEJMoa1105816.

[44] Manfred J Müller, Anja Bosy-Westphal, and Steven B Heymsfield, "Is There Evidence for a Set Point That Regulates Human Body Weight?," *F1000 Medicine Reports* 2 (August 9, 2010), https://doi.org/10.3410/M2-59.

[45] Fung, *The Obesity Code*.

[46] Michael Greger and Gene Stone, *How Not to Die: Discover the Foods Scientifically Proven to Prevent and Reverse Disease*, First edition (New York: Flatiron Books, 2015).

[47] Fung, *The Obesity Code*.

[48] Sareen Annora Stepnick Gropper, Jack L. Smith, and James L. Groff, *Advanced Nutrition and Human Metabolism*, 5th ed (Australia ; United States: Wadsworth/Cengage Learning, 2009).

[49] Hassan Ashfaq Ul et al., "Obesity-Prevent Rather than Cure: Histopathological and Clinical Perspectives," *Journal International Medical Sciences Academy. Vol. 25 No. 3*, no. July-September 2012 (n.d.): 209–10.

[50] Caroline Horizny, "Adipose Tissue and Hormone Regulation," *Taconic Biosciences* (blog), August 22, 2019, https://www.taconic.com/taconic-insights/cardiovascular-disease/adipose-tissue-hormone-regulation.html.

[51] Fung, *The Obesity Code*.

[52] Christine Mikstas, "Brown Fat: What You Need To Know," *Nourish by WebMD* (blog), April 20, 2020, https://www.webmd.com/diet/brown-fat-what-you-need-to-know#1.

[53] Wim Hof, *The Wim Hof Method: Activate Your Full Human Potential* (Boulder, CO: Sounds True, 2020).

[54] "How Inuit Genomes Have Adapted," *Nature* 525, no. 7570 (September 2015): 429–429, https://doi.org/10.1038/525429d.

[55] Guolin Li et al., "Intermittent Fasting Promotes White Adipose Browning and Decreases Obesity by Shaping the Gut Microbiota," *Cell Metabolism* 26, no. 4 (October 2017): 672-685.e4, https://doi.org/10.1016/j.cmet.2017.08.019.

[56] Monoj K. Gupta, "Hydrogenation," in *Practical Guide to Vegetable Oil Processing* (Elsevier, 2017), 171–215, https://doi.org/10.1016/B978-1-63067-050-4.00007-6.

[57] "International Study of Asthma and Allergies in Childhood (ISAAC)," accessed August 4, 2021, http://isaac.auckland.ac.nz/.

[58] "Schädliche Transfette Im Essen Vermeiden," *NDR* (blog), accessed August 6, 2021, https://www.ndr.de/ratgeber/gesundheit/Schaedliche-Transfette-im-Essen-vermeiden,transfett100.html.

[59] Greger and Stone, *How Not to Die*.

[60] Greger and Stone.

[61] "Small Entity Compliance Guide: Trans Fatty Acids in Nutrition Labeling, Nutrient Content Claims, and Health Claims," *FDA* (blog), August 2003, https://www.fda.gov/regulatory-information/search-fda-guidance-documents/small-entity-compliance-guide-trans-fatty-acids-nutrition-labeling-nutrient-content-claims-and.

[62] Greger and Stone, *How Not to Die*.

[63] Werner Bartens, "Kehrtwende in Der Fettecke," *Süddeutsche Zeitung*, November 28, 2013, https://www.sueddeutsche.de/gesundheit/cholesterinsenker-kehrtwende-in-der-fettecke-1.1829749.

[64] Fung, *The Obesity Code*.

[65] T. Colin Campbell and Thomas M. Campbell, *The China Study: The Most Comprehensive Study of Nutrition Ever Conducted and the Startling Implications for Diet, Weight Loss and Long-Term Health*, 1. paperback ed (Dallas, Tex: Benbella Books, 2006).

[66] Giulia Enders, Jill Enders, and David Shaw, *Gut: the inside story of our body's most underrated organ*, 2018.

[67] Greger and Stone, *How Not to Die*.

[68] Greger and Stone.

[69] Fung, *The Obesity Code*.

[70] Peter J. Havel, "Dietary Fructose: Implications for Dysregulation of Energy Homeostasis and Lipid/Carbohydrate Metabolism," *Nutrition Reviews* 63, no. 5 (May 2005): 133–57, https://doi.org/10.1111/j.1753-4887.2005.tb00132.x.

[71] Fung, *The Obesity Code*.

[72] Fung.

[73] Greger and Stone, *How Not to Die*.

[74] Fung, *The Obesity Code*.

[75] "Glycemic Index (GI)," Database, accessed August 26, 2021, https://glycemicindex.com.

[76] Campbell and Campbell, *The China Study*.

[77] Greger and Stone, *How Not to Die*.

[78] Greger and Stone.

[79] Fung, *The Obesity Code*.

[80] Greger and Stone, *How Not to Die*.

[81] Greger and Stone.

[82] Paula Tighe et al., "Effect of Increased Consumption of Whole-Grain Foods on Blood Pressure and Other Cardiovascular Risk Markers in Healthy Middle-Aged Persons: A Randomized Controlled Trial," *The American Journal of Clinical Nutrition* 92, no. 4 (October 1, 2010): 733–40, https://doi.org/10.3945/ajcn.2010.29417.

[83] Greger and Stone, *How Not to Die*.

[84] Greger and Stone.

[85] Bas Kast and Herbert Schäfer, *Der Ernährungskompass Das Fazit aller wissenschaftlichen Studien zum Thema Ernährung - Mit den 12 wichtigsten Regeln der gesunden Ernährung*, 2018, https://nbn-resolving.org/urn:nbn:de:101:1-2018061904025896478482.

[86] Fung, *The Obesity Code*.

[87] Campbell and Campbell, *The China Study*.

[88] Kast and Schäfer, *Der Ernä*.

[89] Campbell and Campbell, *The China Study*.

[90] Kast and Schäfer, *Der Ernä*.

[91] Greger and Stone, *How Not to Die*.

[92] Fung, *The Obesity Code*.

[93] Campbell and Campbell, *The China Study*.

[94] Greger and Stone, *How Not to Die*.

[95] Campbell and Campbell, *The China Study*.

[96] Fung, *The Obesity Code*.

[97] T J Maher and R J Wurtman, "Possible Neurologic Effects of Aspartame, a Widely Used Food Additive.," *Environmental Health Perspectives* 75 (November 1987): 53–57, https://doi.org/10.1289/ehp.877553.

[98] Greger and Stone, *How Not to Die*.

[99] Glenda N. Lindseth et al., "Neurobehavioral Effects of Aspartame Consumption: EFFECTS OF ASPARTAME CONSUMPTION," *Research in Nursing & Health* 37, no. 3 (June 2014): 185–93, https://doi.org/10.1002/nur.21595.

[100] "Additional Information about High-Intensity Sweeteners Permitted for Use in Food in the United States," *FDA* (blog), February 8, 2018, https://www.fda.gov/food/food-additives-petitions/additional-information-about-high-intensity-sweeteners-permitted-use-food-united-states.

[101] Lindseth et al., "Neurobehavioral Effects of Aspartame Consumption."

[102] Fung, *The Obesity Code.*

[103] Martha T. Conklin, Laurel G. Lambert, and Janet B. Anderson, "How Long Does It Take Students to Eat Lunch? A Summary of Three Studies," *The Journal of Child Nutrition & Management. Volume 26, Issue 2*, no. Fall 2002 (n.d.).

[104] R. C. Mollard et al., "Regular Consumption of Pulses for 8 Weeks Reduces Metabolic Syndrome Risk Factors in Overweight and Obese Adults," *British Journal of Nutrition* 108, no. S1 (August 23, 2012): S111–22, https://doi.org/10.1017/S0007114512000712.

[105] T T Shintani et al., "Obesity and Cardiovascular Risk Intervention through the Ad Libitum Feeding of Traditional Hawaiian Diet," *The American Journal of Clinical Nutrition* 53, no. 6 (June 1, 1991): 1647S-1651S, https://doi.org/10.1093/ajcn/53.6.1647S.

[106] Campbell and Campbell, *The China Study.*

[107] Greger and Stone, *How Not to Die.*

[108] Stephanie M. Matt et al., "Butyrate and Dietary Soluble Fiber Improve Neuroinflammation Associated With Aging in Mice," *Frontiers in Immunology* 9 (August 14, 2018): 1832, https://doi.org/10.3389/fimmu.2018.01832.

[109] "U.S. Food and Drug Administration," accessed September 14, 2021, https://www.fda.gov/about-fda/what-we-do.

[110] Greger and Stone, *How Not to Die.*

[111] Omar Benini et al., "Extra-Phosphate Load From Food Additives in Commonly Eaten Foods: A Real and Insidious Danger for Renal Patients," *Journal of Renal Nutrition* 21, no. 4 (July 2011): 303–8, https://doi.org/10.1053/j.jrn.2010.06.021.

[112] Greger and Stone, *How Not to Die.*

[113] Greger and Stone.

[114] Greger and Stone.

[115] Greger and Stone.

[116] Enders, Enders, and Shaw, *Gut.*

[117] Enders, Enders, and Shaw.

[118] Christopher Zoukis, "Vegan Diet Impacts Recidivism," May 20, 2013, https://prisonerresource.com/vegan-diet-impacts-recidivism/.

[119] Enders, Enders, and Shaw, *Gut.*

[120] Enders, Enders, and Shaw.

[121] Enders, Enders, and Shaw.

[122] Enders, Enders, and Shaw.

[123] Riitta Törrönen et al., "Postprandial Glucose, Insulin, and Free Fatty Acid Responses to Sucrose Consumed with Blackcurrants and Lingonberries in Healthy Women," *The American Journal of Clinical Nutrition* 96, no. 3 (September 1, 2012): 527–33, https://doi.org/10.3945/ajcn.112.042184.

[124] Holly L. Nicastro, Sharon A. Ross, and John A. Milner, "Garlic and Onions: Their Cancer Prevention Properties," *Cancer Prevention Research* 8, no. 3 (March 2015): 181–89, https://doi.org/10.1158/1940-6207.CAPR-14-0172.

[125] Roman Leontiev et al., "A Comparison of the Antibacterial and Antifungal Activities of Thiosulfinate Analogues of Allicin," *Scientific Reports* 8, no. 1 (December 2018): 6763, https://doi.org/10.1038/s41598-018-25154-9.

[126] Greger and Stone, *How Not to Die*.

[127] Ankit Goyal et al., "Flax and Flaxseed Oil: An Ancient Medicine & Modern Functional Food," *Journal of Food Science and Technology* 51, no. 9 (September 2014): 1633–53, https://doi.org/10.1007/s13197-013-1247-9.

[128] Greger and Stone, *How Not to Die*.

[129] Hongyu Wu et al., "Association Between Dietary Whole Grain Intake and Risk of Mortality: Two Large Prospective Studies in US Men and Women," *JAMA Internal Medicine* 175, no. 3 (March 1, 2015): 373, https://doi.org/10.1001/jamainternmed.2014.6283.

[130] Mollard et al., "Regular Consumption of Pulses for 8 Weeks Reduces Metabolic Syndrome Risk Factors in Overweight and Obese Adults."

[131] Greger and Stone, *How Not to Die*.

[132] Mir Hadi Seyedzadeh et al., "Study of Curcumin Immunomodulatory Effects on Reactive Astrocyte Cell Function," *International Immunopharmacology* 22, no. 1 (September 2014): 230–35, https://doi.org/10.1016/j.intimp.2014.06.035.

[133] Greger and Stone, *How Not to Die*.

[134] Greger and Stone.

[135] Yafit Hachmo et al., "Hyperbaric Oxygen Therapy Increases Telomere Length and Decreases Immunosenescence in Isolated Blood Cells : A Prospective Trial," *Aging*, November 11, 2020, https://doi.org/10.18632/aging.202188.

[136] Madison Cavanaugh, *The One-Minute Cure: The Secret to Healing Virtually All Diseases* (Beverly Hills, Calif.: Think-outside-the-book Pub., 2008).

[137] Jochen Gartz, *Wasserstoffperoxid - H2O2 das vergessene Heilmittel*, 2015.

[138] Cavanaugh, *The One-Minute Cure.*

[139] Gartz, *Wasserstoffperoxid - H2O2 das vergessene Heilmittel.*

[140] William Campbell Douglass, *Hydrogen Peroxide: Medical Miracle* (Panama: Rhino Publishing, 2003).

[141] Gartz, *Wasserstoffperoxid - H2O2 das vergessene Heilmittel.*

[142] Michael P Lisanti et al., "Hydrogen Peroxide Fuels Aging, Inflammation, Cancer Metabolism and Metastasis: The Seed and Soil Also Needs 'Fertilizer,'" *Cell Cycle* 10, no. 15 (August 2011): 2440–49, https://doi.org/10.4161/cc.10.15.16870.

[143] Claire M. Doskey et al., "Tumor Cells Have Decreased Ability to Metabolize H2O2: Implications for Pharmacological Ascorbate in Cancer Therapy," *Redox Biology* 10 (December 2016): 274–84, https://doi.org/10.1016/j.redox.2016.10.010.

[144] Gartz, *Wasserstoffperoxid - H2O2 das vergessene Heilmittel.*

[145] Douglass, *Hydrogen Peroxide.*

[146] Cavanaugh, *The One-Minute Cure.*

[147] Gartz, *Wasserstoffperoxid - H2O2 das vergessene Heilmittel.*

[148] Cavanaugh, *The One-Minute Cure.*

Made in United States
North Haven, CT
10 November 2026

22088886R00088